Organic Beauty

WITH ESSENTIAL OIL

Over 400+
Homemade Recipes for
Natural Skin Care,
Hair Care, and
Bath & Body Products

Rebecca Park Totilo

Organic Beauty with Essential Oil

Edited by Rachel Park

Typeset by Desy S. (https://www.elance.com/s/coverbook)

Printed in the United States of America.

Published by Rebecca at the Well Foundation, PO Box 60044, St. Petersburg, Florida 33784.
http://RebeccaAtTheWell.org

Disclaimer Notice: The information contained in this book is intended for educational purposes only and is not meant to be a substitute for medical care or prescribe treatment for any specific health condition. Please see a qualified health care provider for medical treatment. We assume no responsibility or liability for any person or group for any loss, damage or injury resulting from the use or misuse of any information in this book. No express or implied guarantee is given regarding the effects of using any of the products described herein.

ISBN 978-0-9827264-2-6

Table of Contents

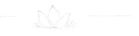

Your Essential Care Guide to Organic Beauty......... 1

Essential Care for the Body 52

Essential Care for the Face 186

Essential Care for the Hair..235

Essential Care for the Mouth 251

Essential Care for the Hands and Nails 272

Essential Care for the Feet..287

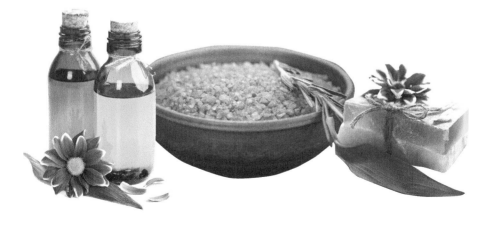

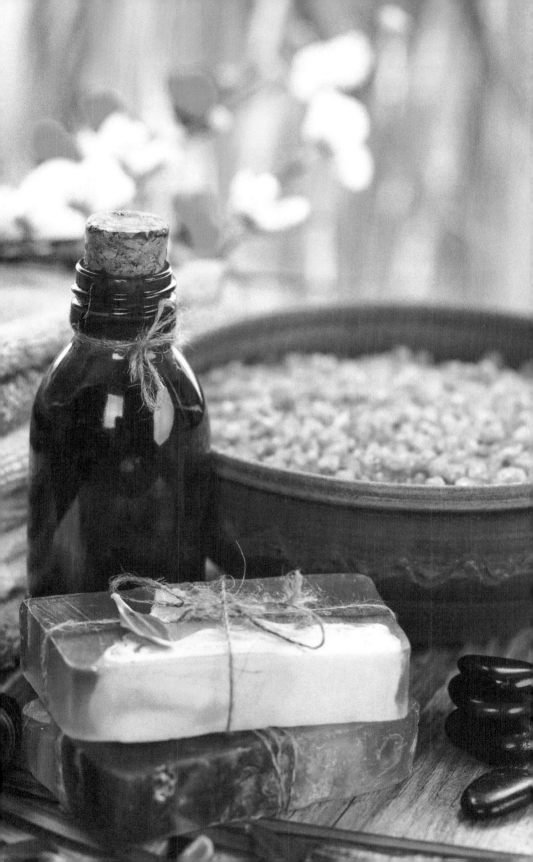

Your Essential Care Guide to Organic Beauty

Every year, Americans spend nearly 50 billion dollars on cosmetic products. The beauty and skin care industry is definitely big business. This includes everything from soaps and gels we use everyday to acne treatments, anti-aging skin products, deodorants, and moisturizers. Each and every year, thousands of new treatments are created and brought to the market, promising to reduce the appearance of aging or energize your body, mind and spirit. There seems to be no end in sight. Unfortunately though, many of these products don't always live up to those promises, simply because man-made ingredients don't possess the same healing properties that nature provides from plants and resins, namely essential oils. In fact, many of the ingredients found in commercial products are dangerous to your health.

We tend to think of our skin, our body's largest organ, as a barrier—keeping environmental toxins from entering our body, protecting us in the winter from the effects of cold, and guarding us in the summer from the ravages of the UV rays of the sun. But it's actually more like a sponge, soaking up everything it comes in contact with.

When you put cosmetics on your skin that are less than healthy—even toxic—all the potentially toxic ingredients are soaked directly into your skin and your system. Surely there must be a better way to make you look and feel better without putting your health on the line everyday! While having healthy skin is far more important than we realize, few of us pay much attention to the commercial products we use to cleanse and moisturize with.

Of course, there's nothing wrong with striving to look as attractive as you can. But at what price are we, as a society, paying for this quest for beauty and youthfulness? According to some health experts, our skin is attacked and stressed every day, being barraged by the myriad of substances we use to clean and repair it, most of which is performed in the name of beauty. Clearly, more than beauty is at stake! As it turns out, the price could very well be our health. Consider this: we're putting substances on our skin that we would never dream of eating.

Are you aware that the U.S. Food and Drug Administration (FDA) has a list that contains some 10,000 cosmetic and skin care ingredients that you can find right now in your bathroom? Most of us take for granted that these products are safe. But more than a whopping 90% of them have never been tested for safety, by the FDA, nor by any other publically accountable institution. In contrast, the European Union has already banned more than 1,000 ingredients used in personal and skin care products. The FDA has only banned ten!

For example, many cosmetics and skin care products such as soap contain a substance called parabens, a fairly common additive that penetrates the skin. Once parabens get into your body, they stay there and slowly damage your system. The FDA estimates that this class of chemical is the most widely used family of preservatives in cosmetics today and is found in 13,200 skin care ingredients. And if you think that the products you're using are parabens-free because they're labeled "organic," think again. Parabens have raised their ugly heads there too. Take a quick look now at the products you are using in your bathroom. Read the labels on your shampoos, your makeup and hair care products, your moisturizers, and even your shaving products. Look for prefixes before this word, like methyl, propyl, butyl and ethyl. These are all types of parabens.

So, just how dangerous could this chemical preservative be? Parabens are linked to a greater risk of breast cancer in women. These substances soak into your skin, linger in your body and then settle into the breast tissue, according to the Women's Community Cancer Project of Cambridge, Massachusetts. Once they're in your system, parabens begin what's called "estrogenic activity." This means they mimic the hormone estrogen and are believed to stimulate breast cancer activity. In a nutshell, the parabens actually fool your body into thinking there's more estrogen present than there really is. In the process, they raise your risk of breast cancer.

So, if brands labeled as "natural" have this dangerous substance lurking inside, how do you avoid this and other potentially dangerous synthetic ingredients? You could become a diligent label reader, but you'd no doubt find there are very few products on the shelves today that are completely natural—despite the advertising hype surrounding them. So how do you avoid these products? The answer is simple: by making your own skin care treatments.

Why Make Your Own Bath & Body Products

There are two reasons for creating your own bath and body products with essential oils to pamper your skin—and believe me you really will feel a wondrous difference from the commercially produced items you've been using!

The first is having peace of mind knowing what is in the products you are using. The products you'll be making call for all-natural ingredients. In fact, many of the ingredients can be found right in your kitchen. This ensures your bath products don't contain any of the harmful and toxic ingredients store-bought products contain, while saving you loads of money. You get to choose which ingredients you want to add—depending on what you have on hand, the possibilities are endless!

But there's a second reason. All commercially derived products containing these complex substances that sound beneficial to your skin such as antioxidants, proteins, vitamins, enzymes, and phytochemicals, are duplicated synthetically. This means they are far less effective than the natural versions. Think of it as taking vitamins versus eating healthy. It's always better to have a good, healthy diet than to rely solely on vitamin tablets—especially synthetic vitamins—for your nourishment.

Ask any professional Aromatherapist and she'll tell you the same thing. The chemical constituents found in essential oils actually work in harmony with your body and have an amazing ability to rejuvenate your skin, unlike synthetics. Essential oil-based treatments are far more effective than the ones the cosmetic companies churn out.

By making your own natural skin care products from the recipes in this book, you will no longer be endangering your health and will still be able to get the results you see advertised on television and in magazines such as:

- Hasten collagen production
- Improve your skin's moisture content
- Boost your skin's ability to protect you from environmental toxins
- Reduce the effects of free radicals that can damage your skin
- Encourage and stimulate the renewal and repair of your skin cells

And, best of all, it doesn't take much time or any fancy equipment. So, where do you start?

This book is a compilation of some of the easiest and most effective skin care therapies around. The recipes are easy to create and all come with years of proven use. Many of these formulas have been handed down for generations from grandmother to mother to daughter. Other recipes were created by professional Aromatherapists who have studied for years and used their knowledge in formulating the most effective remedies for skin care.

You will find recipes for facial scrubs, masks, bath salts, lip balms, body lotions, bath bombs, body oils, body powders, sprays, bubble bath and more! Once you become experienced in creating these easy treatments, you may want to experiment with different essential oils to find the perfect proportions for your personal skin type. This way, your skin can receive the optimum beneficial effects possible.

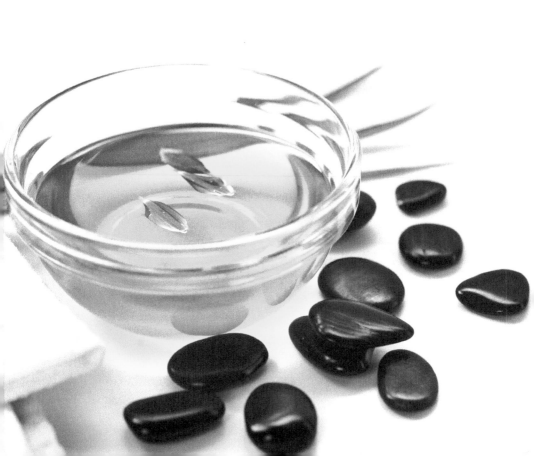

What Are Essential Oils

Essential oils are vital, aromatic fluids distilled from a plant's leaves, flowers, roots, seeds, bark and/or resins. In the case of citrus fruits, these crucial oils are expressed from the fruit's rind.

Considered the essence or lifeblood of the plant, this substance plays an important role in the biological processes of vegetation. The essential oil of a plant serves several functions; their odors attract pollinating insects, while at the same time repelling pests, bacteria, and viruses that can harm the plant. Scientifically, essential oils have been proven to contain the intelligence and vibrational energy of the plant that endows them with the healing power to sustain a plant's life—and people who use essential oils can benefit from the healing power they possess.

It generally takes at least 50 pounds of plant material to make one pound of essential oil (for example, a pound of Rosemary oil requires sixty-six pounds of herbs), but the ratio is sometimes astonishing—it takes 2,300 pounds of Rose flowers to make a single pound of oil!

How Do Essential Oils Work?

Unlike fatty vegetable oils used primarily for cooking, which are composed of molecules too large to penetrate at a cellular level, essential oils are a non-greasy liquid composed of tiny molecules that can penetrate every cell and administer healing at the most fundamental level of our body. Their unique feature allows them to pass through the skin and cell membranes where they are most needed. Because of their structural complexity, essential oils are able to perform multiple functions with just a few drops applied to the skin (in a lotion, cream, or carrier oil).

Since essential oils are derived from a natural plant source, you will notice that the oil does not leave an "oily" or greasy spot. When applied to the skin, they quickly are absorbed and go right to action.

Modern science has attempted to duplicate the chemical constituents and healing capabilities of essential oils, but cannot. Man-made pharmaceuticals lack the intelligence and life-force found in the healing essential oils. In addition, most synthetic duplicates have multiple undesirable side effects—even some that are deadly.

Even though most essential oils have no serious side effects, care should be taken when using them. Please review the section entitled,- *Essential Oil Tips* and safety guidelines before using them. Many people have reported incredible results when using them—however, everyone may not experience the same results as family history, lifestyle, and diet plays a significant role in the body's healing process.

Storage & Care for your Essential Oils

Because essential oils contain no fatty acids, they are not susceptible to rancidity like vegetable oils—but care should be taken to protect them from the degenerative effects of heat, light and air. Store them in tightly sealed, dark glass bottles away from any heat source. When stored properly, your essential oils can maintain their quality for years. (Citrus oils are less stable and should not be stored more than one year after opening.)

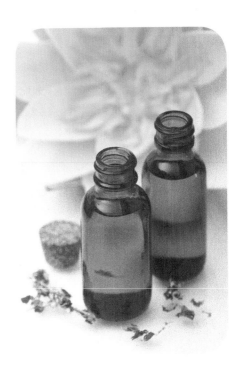

Essential Oil Tips

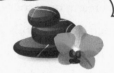

- Always read and follow all label warnings and cautions.
- Keep oils tightly closed and out of the reach of children.
- Always use a vegetable or carrier oil when applying essential oils directly to the skin.
- Skin test oils before using. Dilute a small amount and apply to the skin on your inner arm. If redness, burning, itching, or irritation occurs, stop using the oil immediately.
- For someone who tends to be highly allergic, here is a simple test to use to help determine if he/she is sensitive to a particular oil. First, rub a drop of carrier oil onto the upper chest. In 12 hours, check for redness or other skin irritation. If the skin remains clear, place 1 drop of selected essential oil in 15 drops of the same carrier oil, and again rub into the upper chest. If no skin reaction appears after 12 hours, it's probably safe to use the carrier and essential oil.
- Keep essential oils away from eyes and mucous membranes. If an essential oil gets into the eyes, immediately flush with large quantity of milk and seek medical advice.
- If an essential oil is ingested, rinse mouth out with milk, and then drink a large glass of milk. Seek medical advice immediately.
- If essential oils are splashed onto skin and irritation results, apply carrier oil to the area to dilute.
- Avoid use of these oils during pregnancy: Bitter Almond, Basil, Clary Sage, Clove, Hyssop, Fennel, Juniper, Marjoram, Myrrh, Peppermint, Rose, Rosemary, Sage, Thyme, and Wintergreen.
- These oils may cause irritation to the skin: Allspice, Bitter Almond, Basil, Cinnamon, Clove, Fennel, Fir Needle, Lemon, Lemongrass, Melissa, Peppermint, and Wintergreen.
- Angelica and all citrus oils make the skin more sensitive to ultraviolet light. After applying citrus oils to the skin, avoid exposure to sunlight, since the oils may burn the skin.

Essential Oil Tips (continues)

- Fennel, Hyssop, Sage, and Rosemary should not be used by anyone with epilepsy. People with high blood pressure should avoid Hyssop, Rosemary, Sage, and Thyme.

- Use caution when using essential oils near furniture. It is possible some essential oils will remove the finish. It's best to be careful when handling the bottles.

- Most perfume oils are synthetic and do not offer the therapeutic benefits essential oils do. Even if you only intend on using aromatherapy in your lifestyle for the sheer enjoyment of the aroma, sometimes perfume oils can be harmful. Only pure therapeutic grade essential oils offer healthy benefits.

- Don't buy essential oils with rubber glass dropper tops. Essential oils are very concentrated and will turn the rubber to a gum thus ruining the oil.

- It is also helpful to note the country of origin for the oil. Most good essential oil sellers will readily supply the botanical names and country of origin for the oils that they sell. When comparing one company's oils with another's also pay attention to if either company's oils are organic, wild-crafted, or ethically farmed.

- It is wise not to purchase oils from vendors at street fairs, craft shows, or other limited-time events. Some vendors know beginners have no recourse against them later. This is not to say that there are not highly reputable sellers at such events, but this is a caution for beginners who are not able to reliably judge quality.

- Be selective of where you purchase your essential oils. The quality of essential oils varies widely from company to company. Additionally, some companies may falsely claim that their oils are undiluted or pure when they aren't. It is recommend you purchase your essential oils from http:HealWithEssentialOil.com.

Dilution Chart

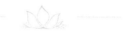

It is important to dilute your essential oil with a suitable carrier oil, so that you can use it on the skin. There are different carrier oils (such as Sweet Almond, Cold-pressed Olive, Flaxseed, Avocado, Grapeseed Extract, and Jojoba) and you will want to select the best one for your purpose and skin type. Carrier oils can be purchased from a natural health food store or grocer, but check labels to make sure the one you select is cold-pressed oil and is suitable for use on the skin.

The following dilution chart shows you the percentage of pure therapeutic essential oil to use to the number of drops of carrier oil (vegetable oil) and will help you convert essential and carrier oil measurements. Use a measuring cup or spoon for carrier oils and pipettes for measuring your essential oils.

For general purposes, the dilution rate for essential oils is generally 2%-3%. For instance, if you use 2-3 drops of pure essential oil, you will dilute by adding about a teaspoon of carrier oil. This should be cut in half for children and senior citizens.

For women who are pregnant, the general rule is a 1% dilution for oils that are safe to use. For a 3.5 ounce bottle (100 ml) carrier oil, add 25 drops essential oil and for 1/3 ounce carrier oil (10 ml or 2 teaspoons), add 2 drops of essential oil.

When you use essential oils for a massage, you will need to dilute with carrier oil. Generally, 2 drops of essential oil should be used per teaspoon of carrier oil (but follow individual recipes if available). A full body massage takes about 1-2 ounces of carrier oil. Any natural carrier oil is fine to use when preparing a massage blend. As a general rule, add

15 drops of essential oil to 30ml of carrier oil. For children and elderly, use only 5-7 drops of essential oil to 30ml of carrier oil.

Two to three drops of essential oils is the most you should use in an eight-hour period. Keep in mind, less is best when it comes to essential oils, and it would be wasteful to use more.

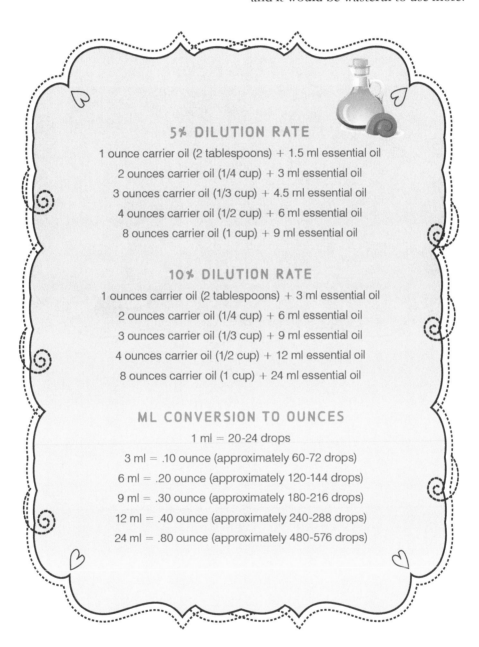

5% DILUTION RATE

1 ounce carrier oil (2 tablespoons) + 1.5 ml essential oil

2 ounces carrier oil (1/4 cup) + 3 ml essential oil

3 ounces carrier oil (1/3 cup) + 4.5 ml essential oil

4 ounces carrier oil (1/2 cup) + 6 ml essential oil

8 ounces carrier oil (1 cup) + 9 ml essential oil

10% DILUTION RATE

1 ounces carrier oil (2 tablespoons) + 3 ml essential oil

2 ounces carrier oil (1/4 cup) + 6 ml essential oil

3 ounces carrier oil (1/3 cup) + 9 ml essential oil

4 ounces carrier oil (1/2 cup) + 12 ml essential oil

8 ounces carrier oil (1 cup) + 24 ml essential oil

ML CONVERSION TO OUNCES

1 ml = 20-24 drops

3 ml = .10 ounce (approximately 60-72 drops)

6 ml = .20 ounce (approximately 120-144 drops)

9 ml = .30 ounce (approximately 180-216 drops)

12 ml = .40 ounce (approximately 240-288 drops)

24 ml = .80 ounce (approximately 480-576 drops)

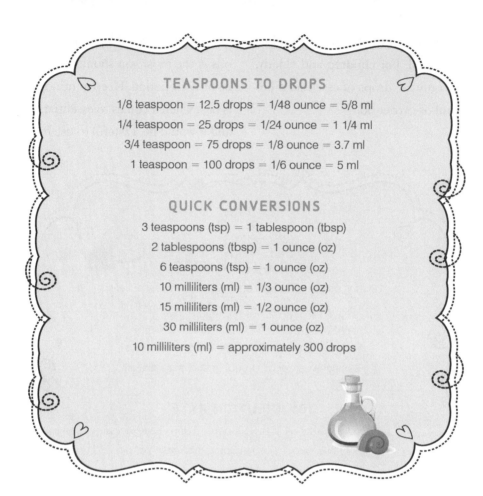

TEASPOONS TO DROPS

1/8 teaspoon = 12.5 drops = 1/48 ounce = 5/8 ml

1/4 teaspoon = 25 drops = 1/24 ounce = 1 1/4 ml

3/4 teaspoon = 75 drops = 1/8 ounce = 3.7 ml

1 teaspoon = 100 drops = 1/6 ounce = 5 ml

QUICK CONVERSIONS

3 teaspoons (tsp) = 1 tablespoon (tbsp)

2 tablespoons (tbsp) = 1 ounce (oz)

6 teaspoons (tsp) = 1 ounce (oz)

10 milliliters (ml) = 1/3 ounce (oz)

15 milliliters (ml) = 1/2 ounce (oz)

30 milliliters (ml) = 1 ounce (oz)

10 milliliters (ml) = approximately 300 drops

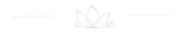

Quick Reference
Blend Chart

This guide quickly shows you how much essential oil to use for each application. For recipes and formulas, be sure to follow amounts listed in the directions. Caution: for children, elderly and pregnant women, please divide essential oil amount in half for body applications.

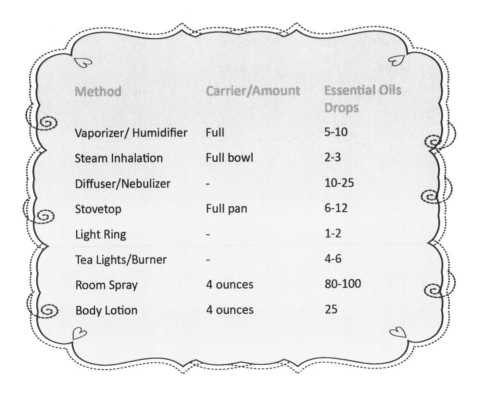

Method	Carrier/Amount	Essential Oils Drops
Vaporizer/ Humidifier	Full	5-10
Steam Inhalation	Full bowl	2-3
Diffuser/Nebulizer	-	10-25
Stovetop	Full pan	6-12
Light Ring	-	1-2
Tea Lights/Burner	-	4-6
Room Spray	4 ounces	80-100
Body Lotion	4 ounces	25

Method	Carrier/Amount	Essential Oils Drops
Body Oil	4 ounces	50
Massage Oil	1 tablespoon	7-10
Shampoo/Conditioner	1 ounce	10
Chest Rub	1 ounce	15-25
Compress	-	8-10
Tissue	-	1-2
Mouthwash	1 teaspoon	2-3
Foot Bath/Spa	Small tub	5
Bath	Full tub	8-10
Shower/Washcloth	Washcloth	1-2
Sauna	1 cup water	1-2
Hot Tub/Jacuzzi	Full	10-15

Methods for Using Essential Oils on the Body

MASSAGE OILS A variety of techniques used in massage therapy can incorporate the use of essential oils. Discover which oils hold the therapeutic properties you find most beneficial and add 7 drops of essential oil per 1 tablespoon of massage oil.

MASSAGE STONES Here's an inexpensive spa treatment you can do at home. Select a flat smooth stone the size of your palm, and heat in the oven at a low temperature until warm. Rub a massage oil blend (10-15 drops of essential oil per 1 ounce of carrier oil) over the heated rock to give your spouse a relaxing massage and penetrate muscles (Himalayan Salt Stones work great for this).

BODY OILS Mix 30 drops of essential oil per 1 ounce of cold-pressed carrier oil, such as Olive oil. Choose an all-purpose oil that smells lovely and is great for muscles, pain, headaches, and tension. As a homemade skin moisturizer for your face, use only 15 drops of essential oil diluted in 2 ounces of carrier oil. Never use more than the suggested quantities—essential oils don't become more effective by using extra, in fact they may have a negative effect.

BODY SPRAYS / FACIAL MISTS Creating your own body sprays and facial mists is one of the easiest ways to use essential oils. For a facial mist, use 8-10 drops of essential oils in a 4-ounce spray bottle filled with distilled water. For body sprays, add 30-40 drops of essential oil per 4-ounce spray bottle filled with distilled water. For room sprays, use 80-100 drops of essential oil per 4-ounce spray bottle with the remainder filled with distilled water. Be careful not to spray in the eyes.

FACIAL STEAM / STEAM INHA-LATION Place 2-3 drops of essential oil in a bowl of hot water. Drape a towel over your head and inhale for 5 minutes. Be careful to use only safe oils, as some essential oils may irritate the eyes. This type of treatment is also beneficial if you are suffering from a cold or upper respiratory ailment.

FACIAL TONERS / ASTRI-NGENTS An important step in your facial skin regime will include using an astringent to remove remaining soap and residue left behind. A simple recipe could include 1/8 cup witch hazel, ¾ cup Rosewater, 1 drop of Cypress essential oil and 2 drops of Sandalwood essential oil.

FACIAL OILS When blending a nourishing essential oil blend for your face, combine 20 drops of essential oil with 2 tablespoons carrier oil. To help you determine which essential oils are best for your skin type, please refer to the chapter entitled, *Essential Oils for the Skin.*

LOTIONS / CREAMS Blending essential oils in an unscented, natural lotion/cream base allows you to benefit from the therapeutic qualities of the essential oil, giving you a non-oily way to apply essential oils. This is particularly beneficial for someone with a skin condition that doesn't do well with oils. The dilution rate for using essential oils in a lotion base is no more than 2%. For adults, use 20 drops of essential oil to 50g of lotion. For children and elderly, use 10 drops of essential oil to 50g of lotion.

BATH / SITZ BATH To help treat problems in the pelvic or genital areas, try adding 5 drops of essential oil in just enough water to cover lower body. For a full bath, add 8-10 drops of essential oil while bath is running. Agitate water in a figure eight motion to make sure the oil is mixed well, preventing irritation to mucous membranes. Another method is to add essential oils after the bath has been drawn. Add essential oils with a palm full of liquid soap or shampoo and swish around to dissolve in the tub. Soak for 15-20 minutes.

BATH SALTS Sea salt is great for distributing essential oils throughout the bath. Use approximately 8-12 drop of essential oils per cup of salt, depending on the strength of the oil. You may want to add more or less, a few drops at a time, depending on your personal preference.

BUBBLE BATH You will need only four main ingredients for homemade bubble bath: glycerin, distilled water, castile soap or unscented shampoo, and essential oils. A good rule of thumb is to use approximately 10-20 drops of essential oils total, depending on how strong each scent is and the health benefits you want, per 1 quart of water and 4 ounces of glycerin and castile soap each.

BODY SCRUBS You will need three essential ingredients in making your homemade scrub: an exfoliant such as sea salt or sugar, or something unique like coffee grounds, seeds, oatmeal or ground nut shell, something to hold it together such as Sweet Almond, Coconut, or Olive oil, and essential oils. Your scrub will consist of half exfoliant and half carrier oil—for example 1 cup sea salt to 1 cup Coconut oil. Add 8-12 drops of essential oils to the blend. If you don't like an oily scrub, you can substitute a gentle body wash for the exfoliant instead. This makes a nice a cleansing scrub, rather than a skin-softening scrub.

SHOWER While showering, add a drop or two of essential oil to a washcloth and rub on body. For shower gels, add 1 ounce of essential oil per every gallon (128oz) of shower gel base, depending upon the strength of the fragrance you choose. Start with ½ ounce of essential oil and slowly add more if you want it stronger. Use only skin-safe essential oils.

COMPRESS Dilute 1 part essential oil with 4 parts carrier oil (Olive oil works great) and apply 8-10 drops on affected area. Using a moist towel or washcloth, cover with a dry towel and leave on for 10 minutes. For inflammation, use a cold compress. If there is no inflammation, use a warm compress.

GARGLE / MOUTHWASH Add 3 drops of essential oil to 1 teaspoon of water to use as a mouthwash. You can make your own mouthwash with 2 drops Peppermint oil, 2 drops Tea Tree oil, ½ teaspoon sea salt and ½ cup warm filtered water.

You can also make your own toothpaste by mixing 3 tablespoons baking soda, 10 drops Tea Tree oil, and 10 drops Peppermint essential oil. Mix all of the ingredients together into a paste then store in a clear glass jar to use up in a week.

Freshen your breath with a drop of Peppermint, Spearmint or Fennel essential oil on the tongue.

MILK BATHS Taking a milk bath will make your skin resilient and soft. These are some of the quickest, easiest homemade bath products you can make. Most recipes call for fresh or powdered milk and softening agents such as baking soda and cornstarch. Use 10-20 drops of essential oils per 2 cups of milk. Adding dried flowers or herbs to enhance the mood, fragrance, and healing properties is a creative option.

BATH SOAPS Essential oils give homemade soap a nice aroma while adding healing properties. A simple recipe for making a nourishing soap includes 4 ounces of castile soap, plus 30-45 drops of your essential oil blend of two to three oils. However, some recipes will call for only 10 drops of essential oils to 4 ounces of glycerin (melt and pour base), depending on the strength of the oil. For cold-press soaps, the SoapQueen. com website recommends using ½ ounce or more of essential oil per pound of oil/fat depending on the fragrance you choose.

BATH BOMBS Bath bombs can be made in an incredible rainbow of colors, spectrum of scents, and in a dizzying assortment of shapes. A combination of acids and bases such as baking soda and Citric acid provide fizzing action, and powdered ingredients such as milk powder, salt, or starch provide filler that acts as a binding agent to keep everything packed tightly. Fragrant essential oils, carrier oil and colorants can be included to add excitement and fun to bath time. For essential oils, use 1%-5% dilution of total weight. For instance, you can add ¼ teaspoon essential oil (or approximately 15 drops) and 1 tablespoon of carrier oil, to a mixture of 1 cup of baking soda, ½ cup of Citric acid, ½ cup cornstarch and ½ cup of Dead Sea Salt.

BATH POWDERS Making your own all-natural bath powder is super simple. Store it in a reusable container that you can refill as needed. A simple recipe for bath powder includes baking soda or arrowroot powder and cornstarch with essential oils added for fragrance and health benefits. Add 10-30 drops of essential oils, depending on your desired scent, per 1 cup of dry ingredients.

LIP BALMS Most lip balm recipes include vegetable oils such as Jojoba, Coconut, Mango butter, and Beeswax, as well as colorant. When making your own lip balms or glosses you can enhance your creation by adding flavor oils or an essential oil like Peppermint. Flavor oils are specifically designed for lip care products by adding scent as well as flavor. Never use a fragrance oil to scent your lip balm since they could irritate your skin or even make you ill. Carefully choose an essential oil that is generally regarded safe for consumption. In addition, make sure it won't cause irritation to this sensitive area of the body. For example, if you want to make enough for 40 lip balm tubes, a simple recipe might call for 1-1 ½ teaspoon of flavor oil or essential oil with 1 ounce Jojoba, 1 ounce fractionated Coconut oil, 2 ounces of Mango butter, and 2 ounces of Beeswax.

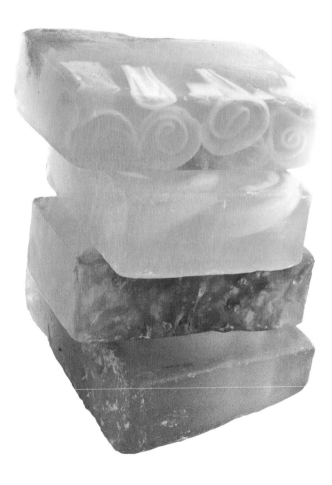

Essential Oils for Setting the Mood

Have you ever noticed when you wake up in the morning and feel sluggish, you suddenly feel invigorated when you smell the aroma of fresh-brewed coffee? Or, how relaxed you feel after a brisk walk in the forest where the scents of spruce, pine, or cedars fill the air? Your homemade bath recipes with essential oils can recreate those feelings and elevate your mood. Even when the scent is too faint to notice healing is taking place. The sense of smell facilitated through the olfactory nerve invites the fragrance of essential oils naturally into the body, simulating the limbic region of the brain (seat of emotions), the pineal gland, and the pituitary gland. The nose, which is wired differently than the other four senses, carries molecules directly into the emotional center of the brain where memories are stored. Because of this, essential oils become a vehicle by which repressed emotions can be released.

Aromatherapy, particularly in the use of pure essential oils, can be extremely useful in promoting strong emotional wellbeing. They can help promote positive emotional states of being and can assist in dealing with issues such as fear, grief, anger, or frustration.

Refer to the list below when you are looking to create or enhance a certain mood with essential oils in your bath and body recipes:

PEACEFUL Lavender, Sandalwood, Honeysuckle, Roman Chamomile, Ylang Ylang, Rose, Lemon Verbena, Orange, Patchouli, Blue Tansy, Bergamot, Clary Sage, Niaouli, Frankincense, Geranium, Cedarwood, Onycha (Benzoin), Jasmine, Tangerine, Neroli, and Marjoram.

RELAXING Lavender, Sandalwood, Roman Chamomile, Ylang Ylang, Tangerine, Rose, Lemon Verbena, Patchouli, Bergamot, Clary Sage, Geranium, Onycha (Benzoin), Jasmine, Neroli, Marjoram, Melissa, Petitgrain, Citronella, and Yarrow.

ENERGIZING Rosemary, Peppermint, Lemon, Lime, Balsam Pine, Orange, Thyme, Jasmine, Myrrh, Cardamom, Bergamot, Cypress, Marjoram, and Eucalyptus.

STIMULATING & INVIGORATING Bergamot, Orange, Rosemary, Lemon Verbena, Spearmint, Sage, Pine, Cypress, Ginger, Grapefruit, Clary Sage, Lemon, Basil, Frankincense, Patchouli, Black Pepper, Wintergreen, and Sandalwood.

MENTAL CLARITY Frankincense, Peppermint, Rosemary, Grapefruit, Lemon, Lemongrass, Roman Chamomile, Cinnamon, Orange, Bergamot, Black Pepper, Basil, Eucalyptus, Vetiver, and Ylang Ylang.

FOCUS & CONCENTRATION Lemon, Fennel, Thyme, Grapefruit, Bergamot, Basil, Cypress, Cinnamon, Peppermint, Cedarwood, Lemongrass, Eucalyptus, and Nutmeg.

ROMANTIC & EXOTIC Ylang Ylang, Rose, Jasmine, Cassia, Cinnamon, Sandalwood, Orange, Vanilla, Bergamot, Neroli, and Patchouli.

JOYFUL & HAPPY Orange, Rose, Jasmine, Ginger, Clove, Cinnamon, Sandalwood, Frankincense, Lemon, Bergamot, Lime, Grapefruit, and Petitgrain.

POSITIVE & CONFIDENT Cypress, Fennel, Ginger, Grapefruit, Jasmine, Orange, Basil, Lemon, Myrrh, Patchouli, Geranium, Frankincense, and Pine.

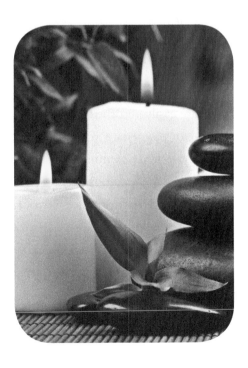

Essential Oils for the Skin

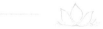

Most of today's skin care products contain harmful petrochemicals that can cause skin irritation or allergic reactions. This is why so many women are turning back to nature and looking for alternatives when caring for their skin. With skin being the largest organ of our body, it makes sense to care for it with what nature provides in pure extracts from plants versus chemical additives and preservatives. Essential oils are easily absorbed into the skin and can oxygenate your skin and rehydrate your complexion. While treating skin conditions, essential oils in your homemade products not only promote wellness but also enhance beauty. Essential oils are particularly useful for regenerating skin cells that has suffered damage from accidents, surgery, or other scarring. Essential oils can speed healing time, reduce or eliminate scars, and even greatly diminish the appearance of old ones. For best results, refer to this handy reference guide to see which essential oils are suitable for your skin type to help you keep (or get back) that youthful glow.

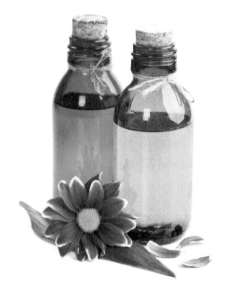

ANGELICA: has a peppery, rich, herbal, earthy, woody and musk animal odor. In Chinese medicine it is used to relieve cramps, infrequent and irregular periods, PMS, and ease menopausal symptoms. May be anti-spasmodic, carminative, depurative, diaphoretic, digestive, diuretic, hepatic, stomachic and tonic; however, it has photosensitizing properties as well, as a nervine stimulant. Angelica essential oil is considered generally non-toxic and non-irritant; however it is known to be phototoxic. After any application to the skin, avoid direct exposure to strong sunlight for up to 12 hours. Avoid use during pregnancy.

ANISE SEED: has a spicy-sweet aroma; because of its high anethole content, Anise Seed is considered to have antiseptic, anti-spasmodic, carminative, diuretic, and expectorant properties. Additionally, it is reputed to control lice and itch mite. This oil is very potent and should not to be used on sensitive skin. Avoid use during pregnancy.

BASIL: is used to relieve muscular aches and pains, colds and flu, hay fever, asthma, bronchitis, mental fatigue, anxiety, and depression; it is very soothing and uplifting, and is popular with massage therapists for alleviating tension and stress in their patients. When applied in dilution, Basil is reputed to be a good insect repellent, while the linalool's mild analgesic properties are known to help to relieve insect bites and stings. May irritate sensitive skin. Avoid use during pregnancy.

BERGAMOT: is used in many skin care creams and lotions because of its refreshing and citrus nature. It is ideally suited to help calm inflamed skin, and is an ingredient in some creams for eczema and psoriasis. Its chemical makeup has antiseptic properties, which help ward off infection and aid recovery. It is a favorite oil of Aromatherapists in treating depression. Bergamot essential oil has phototoxic properties and exposure to the sun must be avoided after use. It may also interfere with the action of certain prescription drugs.

BIRCH: has a sweet, sharp, camphoraceous scent that is very fresh and similar to Wintergreen; is credited with being analgesic, anti-inflammatory, anti-rheumatic, antiseptic, astringent, depurative, diuretic and tonic. It is an effective addition to many massage oil blends for sore muscles, sprains and painful joints because of these anti-inflammatory and antispasmodic properties. Birch essential oil is potentially toxic and may cause skin irritation. Use in dilution and avoid during pregnancy.

BLUE TANSY: has a surprisingly sweet scent making it perfect for applications in skin care products and skin therapies. Blue Tansy contains the active azulene, best known for its skin care properties and as an anti-inflammatory agent. It has been credited by Aromatherapists as being an antihistamine and antispasmodic. It is believed to induce relaxation, reduce nervous tension and stress, and is beneficial for allergies as a stimulant for the thymus gland. Special attention should be given to its blue color as it may change cream or lotion colors. Tansy Blue Essential Oil is generally non-irritating and non-toxic. Avoid use during pregnancy.

CAJEPUT: has a fresh, camphoraceous aroma with a slight fruity note. It has antiseptic and anti-microbial properties, which make it used chiefly as a local application for skin ailments. Other properties include analgesic, anti-neuralgic, antispas-

modic, and insecticidal assets. No known toxicity. Avoid during pregnancy.

CAMPHOR, WHITE: is the preferred grade in scenting detergents, soaps, disinfectants, deodorants, room sprays and other household products. In aromatherapy, Camphor is known to be clarifying, energizing, and purifying. Camphor oil is powerful oil and should be used with care. Overdosing can cause convulsions and vomiting. Pregnant women or persons suffering from epilepsy and asthma should not use it.

CARDAMOM: is an antispasmodic tonic and uplifting oil. Commonly used in aromatherapy as a tonic for the stomach, heartburn, digestive and dyspepsia related remedies; it contains cineole, which helps break up chest congestion while boosting the immune system. Cardamom is also helpful for muscle cramps, catarrh, sinus headache and physical exhaustion. It is best used in baths, massage oils, lotions and in a diffuser. For the body, its stimulating nature warms sore muscles and supports circulation; for the mind, it improves mental clarity and uplifts one's spirit. Cardamom is known to warm the heart, with a long history of being used as an aphrodisiac. Non-toxic, non-irritant and non-sensitizing. Avoid use during pregnancy.

CARROT SEED: is considered one of the best oils to enhance the appearance of mature skin; stimulates cell growth while removing toxins, giving the skin a more toned, youthful appearance; useful in treating scars, wounds and burns. Non-toxic, non-irritant and non-sensitizing. Avoid use during pregnancy.

CASSIA: has antiseptic properties, killing various types of bacteria and fungi; it is a dermal irritant, dermal sensitizer and a mucus membrane irritant and should be avoided in pregnancy.

CEDARWOOD: assists with acne, arthritis, dandruff, and dermatitis; it is used in commercial soaps, cosmetics and perfumes, especially men's colognes. Non-toxic, non-irritant. Avoid during pregnancy.

CHAMOMILE, GERMAN: acts as a relaxing and rejuvenating agent; calms nerves, reduces stress and aids with insomnia; contains excellent anti-inflammatory and antibiotic properties that can assist with cuts,

wounds and insect bites; is an excellent skin cleanser. Good for dry and itchy skin, eases puffiness and strengthens tissues; smoothes out broken capillaries thus improving skin elasticity. Non-toxic, nonirritant, causes dermatitis in some individuals. Do not use the essential oil during pregnancy because it is a uterine stimulant. Also, this oil should not be used by someone who has an allergy to ragweed.

CHAMOMILE, ROMAN: effective for skin care (for most skin types), acne, allergies, boils, burns, eczema, inflamed skin conditions, wounds, menstrual pain, premenstrual syndrome, headache, insomnia, and nervous tension; it is used commercially in shampoos for fair hair as it can lighten hair color. Non-toxic and non-irritant. It should be avoided during pregnancy. Also, this oil should not be used by anyone who has an allergy to ragweed.

CINNAMON: contains antiseptic and antimicrobial properties with its pleasant scent, and is considered a perfect additive to creams, lotions, and soaps. Used by the ancient Egyptians for foot massages and in love potions; can cause irritation to the skin and mucous membranes—particularly in large doses. Can be irritating to the skin and mucous membranes - particularly in large doses; sensitizing must be kept in mind when treating a client. It should always be used in dilution. Avoid use during pregnancy.

CITRONELLA: is an antiseptic, deodorant, insecticide, tonic and a stimulant; commonly used for its insecticidal and bug-repellent properties; it is used in soaps and candles, and has applications in massage to help with minor infections and combating colds and flu; can be used for excessive perspiration and for conditioning oily skin and hair; may irritate sensitive skin and can be sensitizing to those with hay fever. Avoid use during pregnancy.

CLARY SAGE: can be used as a deodorant, antidepressant, and sedative; used as an agent to clean greasy hair; it is non-toxic, and non-sensitizing. This is a great oil for acne and does a wonderful job with wrinkles and fine lines. Clary Sage Oil is non-toxic, and non-sensitizing. Do not use during pregnancy.

CLOVE: has a spicy and rich scent; effective agent for minor aches and pains, particularly dental pain because of its numerous effects on oral tissues; can cause sensitization in some individuals and should be used in dilution. Avoid use during pregnancy.

CORIANDER: works as an analgesic, aphrodisiac, antispasmodic, carminative, deodorant, fungicidal, and is revitalizing and stimulating; relieves mental fatigue, migraine pain, tension and nervous weakness; its warming effect is helpful for alleviating pain such as rheumatism, arthritis and muscle spasms.

CYPRESS: is used to combat excessive perspiration, particularly in the feet; it is used for hemorrhoids, oily skin, rheumatism, and varicose veins. This very relaxing oil has the properties of an astringent and has been used in skin care applications. This oil is regarded as being very gentle and suitable for all skin types.

EUCALYPTUS: is used on all sorts of skin ailments such as burns, blisters, wounds, insect bites, lice, and skin infections; used to combat the effects of colds and flu, and great for sore muscles and joints; should be used in dilution, and avoided during pregnancy. It is considered toxic if taken internally, non-irritant and non-sensitive. Avoid if you have high blood pressure or epilepsy.

FENNEL: is credited with being carminative, depurative, diuretic, expectorant, laxative, stimulant; it is also believed to be invigorating, restoring, stimulating, and warming; is used in soap-making and cosmetics. This product may cause photosensitivity and contact dermatitis. May cause skin irritation. Dilute well before use. Avoid use during pregnancy.

FIR NEEDLE: is a popular oil used in men's fragrances, bath preparations, air fresheners, herbal oils, soaps, and shaving creams. It is non-toxic, non-irritant and non-sensitizing. Do not use this oil undiluted, or topically without using a patch test first, as it may cause contact dermatitis. Liquid may cause irritation to the eyes. Avoid use during pregnancy.

FRANKINCENSE: is highly prized in the perfumery and aromatherapy industry; it is widely used in skin care products' manufacturing as it is considered a valuable ingredient having remarkable anti-aging, rejuvenating and healing properties. Frankincense

essential oil is non-toxic, non-irritant and non-sensitizing. Avoid use during pregnancy.

GALBANUM: is used externally as a poultice for inflammatory swelling, along with Frankincense and Myrrh in baths, and in making perfume oils and cosmetics; is non-toxic, non-irritant and non-sensitizing. Use well diluted and avoid during pregnancy.

GERANIUM: is used as an astringent, haemostatic, diuretic, antiseptic, anti-spasmodic and as an anti-infectious agent; great all-over balancing effect on the skin, creating a balance between oily and dry skin; wards off mosquitoes and head lice. This oil works wonders for wrinkles and is also indicated for disturbed and sensitive skin, as well as broken capillaries; is a good overall skin cleanser. Wonderful oil for mature and troubled skin and brings a radiant glow and promotes circulation. Geranium is well tolerated by most individuals, but since it helps in balancing the hormonal system, care must be taken during pregnancy.

GINGER: is good for colds and flu, nausea (motion sickness, morning sickness), rheumatism, coughs and circulation issues; it has warming properties that help to relieve muscular cramps, spasms, and aches; eases stiffness in joints; can irritate sensitive skin. Avoid use during pregnancy.

GRAPEFRUIT: is spiritually uplifting, eases muscle fatigue and stiffness; eases nervous exhaustion and relieves depression; it also helps purify congested, oily and acne prone skin; it is sometimes added to creams and lotions as a natural toner and cellulite treatment; can cause photosensitivity; Avoid use during pregnancy.

HELICHRYSUM: is effective for acne, bruises, boils, burns, cuts, dermatitis, eczema, irritated skin and wounds; it supports the body through post-viral fatigue and convalescence, and can also be used to repair skin damaged by psoriasis, eczema or ulceration; it is non-toxic, non-irritating and non-sensitizing. Avoid use during pregnancy.

HYSSOP: is anti-rheumatic, antiseptic, antispasmodic, carminative, diuretic, sedative, stimulant, a tonic and as a vulnerary agent; historically, Hyssop was referred to in the Bible for its cleansing effect in connection with plague, leprosy and chest ailments; used for purification to ward off lice. Organic Hyssop Essential Oil is non-irritant, non-sensitizing but does contain pinocamphone and should be used in moderation. Avoid use during pregnancy and by people suffering from epilepsy.

JASMINE: is well respected for its aphrodisiac properties; it is a sensual, soothing, calming oil that promotes love and peace. It is important to note that all absolutes are extremely concentrated by nature; the complexity of the fragrance, particularly the rare and exotic notes, is well regarded as an aphrodisiac, though it is also considered an antidepressant, sedative, and antispasmodic.

JUNIPER: is supportive, restoring, and a tonic aid; used in acne treatments and for oily skin as well as dermatitis, weeping eczema, psoriasis, and blocked pores; considered to be purifying and clearing; is non-irritating and non-sensitizing. Returns skin tissue to normal functioning. Juniper Berry Essential Oil is non-irritating and non-sensitizing. Avoid use during pregnancy.

LAVENDER: is most commonly used for burns and the healing of skin; it has antiseptic and analgesic properties that will ease pain of a burn and prevent infection; it also has cytophylactic properties that promote rapid healing and helps reduce scarring. Lavender does an excellent job at balancing oil production in the skin as well as clearing blemishes and evening skin tone. It's indicated for all skin types and even helps to hydrate dry skin. Lavender can be used at any step in your skin care regimen. Lavender French Essential Oil is non-toxic, non-irritating and non-sensitizing.

LEMON: is recognized as a cleanser and antiseptic with refreshing and cooling properties. On skin and hair it can be used for its cleansing effect, as well as for treating cuts and boils; is non-toxic, but may cause skin irritation for some. Lemon is also phototoxic and should be avoided prior to exposure to direct sunlight. Avoid use during pregnancy.

LEMONGRASS: is known for its invigorating and antiseptic properties; can be used in facial toners as its astringent properties help fight acne and greasy skin; an excellent anti-depressant, Lemongrass tones and fortifies the nervous system and can be used in bath for soothing muscular nerves and pain; it has a great reputation for keeping insects away. Avoid in glaucoma and with children. Use caution in prostatic hyperplasia and with skin hypersensitivity or damaged skin. Avoid use during pregnancy.

LEMON MYRTLE: is an extremely potent antibacterial and germicide; a much more effective germ killer than Tea Tree. Avoid use during pregnancy.

LIME: has a crisp, refreshing citrus scent with uplifting and revitalizing properties; it acts as an astringent on skin where it helps clear oily skin. Lime is considered phototoxic. Users should avoid direct sunlight after application. Avoid use during pregnancy.

MANDARIN: is often used as a digestive aid and to ease anxiety; is commonly used in soaps, cosmetics, perfumes and colognes. It also has many applications in the flavoring industry; may be phototoxic. Direct sunlight should be avoided after use. Avoid use during pregnancy.

MARJORAM: is a comforting oil; can be massaged into the abdomen during menstruation, or added to a warm compress; useful for treating tired aching muscles or in a sports massage; can be added to a warm/hot bath at the first signs of a cold. It can also be used in masculine, oriental, and herbal-spicy perfumes and colognes. Marjoram is generally non-toxic, non-irritating and non-sensitizing. Avoid use during pregnancy.

MYRRH: is characterized as anti-microbial, antifungal, astringent, healing, tonic, stimulant, carminative, expectorant, diaphoretic, locally antiseptic, immune stimulant, bitter, circulatory stimulant, anti-inflammatory, and antispasmodic. Myrrh can be possibly toxic in high concentrations, and should not be used during pregnancy.

MYRTLE: is used as an astringent, antiseptic, vulnerary, bactericidal, expectorant and as a decongestant; used to combat sore throats and coughs. Myrtle can be possibly toxic in high concentrations, and should not be used during pregnancy.

NEROLI: increases circulation and stimulates new cell growth; it prevents scarring and stretch marks, and is useful in treating skin conditions linked to emotional stress; any type of skin can benefit from this oil, although it is particularly good for dry, irritated or sensitive skin; it regulates oiliness and minimizes enlarged pores; helps clear acne and blemished skin, especially if the skin lacks moisture; with regular treatment, it can reduce the appearance of fragile or broken capillaries and varicose veins. This oil is non-toxic and non-sensitizing. Avoid use during pregnancy. Useful for dry, sensitive and mature skin as it helps improves elasticity.

NIAOULI: is an analgesic, anti-rheumatic, antiseptic, anti-spasmodic, stimulant; used locally for a wide variety of ailments including aches and pains, respiratory conditions, cuts and infections; it is also used to purify water. Due to its powerful antiseptic qualities it's a good choice of oil to treat skin conditions such as acne, boils, burns, cuts, insect bites and other similar conditions; is used in pharmaceutical preparations such as gargles, cough drops, toothpastes, and mouth sprays. Niaouli is non-toxic and non-sensitizing. Avoid use during pregnancy.

NUTMEG: is used as a treatment for arthritis, fatigue, muscle aches, poor circulation, and rheumatism; it is a valuable addition to many aromatherapy blends, adding warmth, spice and inspiration, when used in very small amounts. Nutmeg can be used in soaps, candle making, dental products and hair lotions. If used in large amounts, it can cause toxic symptoms such as nausea and tachycardia. Avoid use during pregnancy.

ONYCHA (BENZOIN): has a sweet, warm, vanilla-like aroma; its main constituent is benzoic acid, which has properties that are antiseptic, anti-depressant, anti-inflammatory, carminative, deodorant, diuretic and expectorant. The sweet resin is widely used as a fixative in perfumes but has also been used medicinally for respiratory ailments and skin conditions such as acne, eczema and psoriasis. Benzoin is a non-toxic and non-irritant, but a mild sensitizer and should be avoided if you have allergy-prone skin.

ORANGE: works as an antidepressant, antiseptic, antispasmodic, aphrodisiac, carminative, deodorant, stimulant (nervous) and tonic (cardiac, circulatory); it helps with dull skin, the flu, gums, and stress; is considered phototoxic and exposure to sunlight should be avoided. Do not use if pregnant.

OREGANO: is considered nature's cure-all due to high carvacol and thymol content; potent antiviral, antifungal, antibacterial and anti-parasitic properties; in topical applications can be used to treat itches, skin infections, cuts and wounds; its anti-inflammatory properties makes it effective against swelling and pain caused by rheumatism; can be used as a fragrance component in soaps, colognes and perfumes, especially men's fragrances; Oregano is both a dermal irritant and a mucous membrane irritant. Avoid use during pregnancy.

PALMAROSA: is used as an antiseptic, bactericidal, hydrating, stimulant (circulatory), and tonic; used extensively as a fragrance component in cosmetics, perfumes and especially soaps due to its excellent tenacity; great as a disinfectant. Palmarosa is effective in treating acne surface scars and wrinkles caused by long exposure to the sun. It delivers exceptional hydration to the skin and some research demonstrates its ability to renew skin cells and assist in the regulation of sebum production. Palmarosa is a dermal irritant. Avoid use during pregnancy.

PARSLEY: works as an antiseptic, astringent, carminative, and diuretic; on the skin, it helps clear bruises, is a tonic to the scalp and kills head lice; is widely used in soaps, detergents, cosmetics, and men's colognes; moderately toxic and irritating; use in dilution. Avoid use during pregnancy.

PATCHOULI: is effective for combating nervous disorders, helping with dandruff, sores, skin irritations and acne; specific properties include use as an antidepressant, anti-inflammatory, antimicrobial, antiseptic, antitoxic, antiviral, aphrodisiac, astringent, bactericidal, deodorant, diuretic, fungicidal, nerving, prophylactic, stimulating and tonic agent; has been shown to stimulate cell regeneration. It is excellent for mature, dry, and chapped skin. In the perfumery industry, Patchouli improves with age, and the aged product is what is preferred over freshly harvested; in aromatherapy, it is an excellent fixative that can help extend other, more expensive oils. No cautions.

PEPPER, BLACK: is used in the treatment of pain, rheumatism, chills, flu, colds, poor circulation, exhaustion, muscular aches; it is analgesic, antiseptic, anti-spasmodic, anti-toxic, aphrodisiac, digestive, and diuretic; may cause irritation to sensitive skin and if used too much could over-stimulate the kidneys. Avoid use during pregnancy due to its possible skin sensitizing effect.

PEPPERMINT: has long been credited as being useful in combating stomach ailments. It is viewed as an antispasmodic and antimicrobial agent. Most people know it as a flavoring or scenting agent in food, beverages, skin and hair care products (where it has a cooling effect by constricting capillaries and helping with bruises and sore joints), as well as soaps and candles. Peppermint can be sensitizing due to the menthol content. Avoid use during pregnancy.

PETITGRAIN: is believed to have uplifting properties; used in the skin care industry for acne, oily skin, and as a deodorizing agent. Petitgrain is generally non-toxic, non-irritant, non-sensitizing. Avoid use during pregnancy.

PINE: is viewed as an analgesic, antibacterial, antibiotic, anti-fungal, antiseptic, and antiviral; good as a circulatory agent, decongestant and deodorant. It has been applied to eczema, cuts, lice, muscular aches, neuralgia, psoriasis, rheumatism, ringworm, scrapes, and sinusitis; is considered safe since it is non-toxic and non-irritant, but should be used with care on the skin since it can cause irritation in high dosage and may sensitize the skin.

ROSE: is an uplifting aphrodisiac; is great for meditation. This product is very common in perfumery; it's a good emollient and excellent for skin preparation. Particularly good for mature, dry, or sensitive skin; as a tonic it has a soothing quality for inflammation and constricting action on capillaries. Avoid use during the first trimester of pregnancy.

ROSE GERANIUM: has the ability to both uplift and sedate; works wonders for the emotions; great for skin care and can help in the treatment of acne, bruises, burns, cuts, dermatitis, eczema, hemorrhoids, lice, mosquito repellent, ringworm, ulcers, edema, poor circulation, PMS, menopausal problems, stress and neuralgia; tra-ditionally used as an astringent; used in perfumery and the cosmetics industry as it can be made to imitate many fragrances and is often used to "stretch" the much more expensive oil of Rose; Rose Geranium is non-toxic, non-irritant and generally non-sensitizing, though it can cause sensitivity in some people since it balances the hormonal system. Avoid use during pregnancy.

ROSEMARY: stimulates cell renewal; it improves dry or mature skin, eases lines and wrinkles, and heals burns and wounds. It can also clear acne, blemishes or dull dry skin by fighting bacteria and regulating oil secretions. It improves circulation and can reduce the appearance of broken capillaries and varicose veins; tones and tightens the skin and is helpful for sagging skin. Rosemary helps to overcome mental fatigue and sluggishness by stimulating and strengthening the entire nervous system; enhances mental clarity while aiding alertness and concentration. It can help you cope with stressful conditions and gain clarity; is generally non-toxic and non-sensitizing but is not suitable for people with epilepsy or high blood pressure. Avoid use during pregnancy.

ROSE OF SHARON (LABDANUM): is anti-microbial, antiseptic, astringent and expectorant; it acts as a fixative in perfumes and is widely used in the perfumery industry. It is also considered useful in skin care preparations especially for mature skin and wrinkles; is generally non-toxic and non-sensitizing. Avoid use during pregnancy.

ROSEWOOD: is credited with being a bactericidal, anti-fungal, anti-viral, anti-parasitic cellular stimulant, immune system stimulant, tissue regenerator, tonic, antidepressant, antimicrobial, and as an aphrodisiac. It is also regarded as a general balancer to the emotions. Rosewood is rich in linalool, a chemical that can be transformed into a number of derivatives of value to the flavor and fragrance industries. The oil is antibacterial and very effective in relieving skin irritations and blemishes. It is also effective in maintaining the skin's oil balance and elasticity. Avoid use during pregnancy. It is a possible irritant to sensitive skin.

SAGE: is used as an anti-inflammatory, antiseptic and astringent. In aromatherapy, it is believed to calm the nerves, assist with grief and depression and also assist with female sterility as well as menopausal problems. For topical applications, Sage is reputed to ease swelling, relieve pain caused by rheumatism; and it may be used to reduce pore size, heal wounds and infections, and assist with skin conditions such as psoriasis and dermatitis. It is an oral toxin and should not be used during pregnancy, or by persons suffering from epilepsy or high blood pressure.

SANDALWOOD: creates an exotic, sensual mood with a reputation as an aphrodisiac; used extensively in the perfume industry as a fixative and in body care products for the fragrance it provides. In aromatherapy, Sandalwood is used to help combat bronchitis, chapped and dry skin, mood disturbances, stress and stretch marks. It is said to have antimicrobial properties which makes it effective in treating skin conditions such as acne, oily skin and eczema; it is good for dehydrated skin. It is a powerful antibacterial and anti-fungal agent.

Sandalwood is considered non-toxic, non-irritant and non-sensitizing.

SPEARMINT: is used as a local/topical anesthetic, antispasmodic, astringent, carminative, decongestant, digestive, diuretic, expectorant, stimulant and restorative; it is an uplifting oil, great for alleviating fatigue and depression. It is also reputed to relieve itching (pruritis, eczema, urticaria), cools the skin and aids in healing of wounds, sores and scabs. Spearmint may irritate mucous membranes. Avoid use during pregnancy.

SPIKENARD: is used by Aromatherapists for rashes, wrinkles, cuts, insomnia, migraines, and wounds. Spikenard should be avoided during pregnancy.

SPRUCE: is used for treatments of asthma, bronchitis, coughs, colds, flu, infection, muscle aches and pains, poor circulation, and respiratory weakness; it is believed to be a spiritual oil. Spruce should be avoided during pregnancy. At low doses it is non-toxic, non-irritating, and non-sensitizing.

TANGERINE: is refreshing and rejuvenating; its aroma clears the mind and can help to eliminate emotional confusion; it is very comforting, soothing and warming; used in perfumes, soaps, and as an antispasmodic, carminative, digestive, diuretic, sedative, stimulant (digestive and lymphatic), and tonic agent. Tangerine is similar to other essential oils in the citrus family in that it can be phototoxic and skin should not to expose to sunlight after a treatment. Similarly, the oil should be diluted well before use on the skin. Avoid use during pregnancy.

TEA TREE: is best known as a very powerful immune stimulant; it helps fight all three categories of infectious organisms (bacteria, fungi, and viruses); used in vapor therapy, Tea Tree can help with colds, measles, sinusitis and viral infections. For skin and hair, it has been used to combat acne, oily skin, head lice and dandruff. It is wonderful for spot treating, clears up pimples and greatly reduces their reoccurrence due to its antimicrobial and anti-inflammatory power. Tea Tree may cause dermal sensitization in some people. Do not take internally.

THYME: has antiseptic qualities and is stimulating, uplifting, and reviving. Thyme is a possible skin irritant. It can be toxic if not properly diluted. Avoid use during pregnancy.

TURMERIC: is viewed as a strong relaxant and balancer. It has historical applications as an antiseptic aid for skin care use against acne and facial hair in women. Turmeric has potential irritating and toxic effects when used in large concentrations. Avoid use during pregnancy.

VALERIAN: is used to combat insomnia, nervousness, restlessness, tension, agitation, headaches as the result of nervous tension, and panic attacks. It has also been used on muscle spasms, palpitations of the heart, cardiovascular spasm and neuralgia. Valerian is believed to be a suitable replacement for catnip based on similar chemical components; it is gaining popularity as a natural alternative to commercially available sedatives. It has possible skin sensitizing properties; is non-toxic and non-irritating at low doses. Avoid use during pregnancy and around children.

VANILLA: is considered a premiere sensual aphrodisiac and one of the most popular flavors/aromas; it is comforting and relaxing and is a popular ingredient in oriental-type perfumes. No known toxicity. Avoid high concentration in pregnancy. It may change the color in soaps and body care products. Avoid very high concentrations in skin care.

VETIVER: is believed to be deeply relaxing and comforting. It is used as a base note in perfumery and aromatherapy applications. No known toxicity. Avoid high concentration in pregnancy.

WINTERGREEN: serves as an antiseptic, diuretic, stimulant, emenagogue and anti- rheumatic; very useful in rheumatic conditions and helps with muscular pains; particularly good for athletes. Avoid use during pregnancy. Safety with young children, nursing women, or those with severe liver or kidney disease is not known.

YARROW: is credited with having an energy similar to that of the earth; balancing, uplifting oil with practical applications on gynecological issues, wounds and open sores; used in cosmetics for dry skin care. Yarrow has no known toxicity and is non-irritant in low concentration.

YLANG YLANG: assists with problems such as high blood pressure, rapid breathing and heartbeat, nervous conditions, as well as impotence and frigidity; is best suited for use in the perfumery and skin care industries. Has a balancing effect on sebum and is useful for both oily and dry skin types. Ylang Ylang can cause sensitivity in some people and excessive use of it may lead to headaches and nausea.

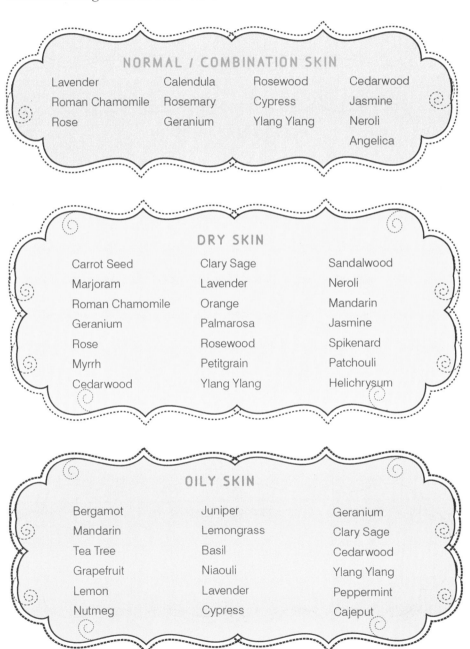

NORMAL / COMBINATION SKIN

Lavender	Calendula	Rosewood	Cedarwood
Roman Chamomile	Rosemary	Cypress	Jasmine
Rose	Geranium	Ylang Ylang	Neroli
			Angelica

DRY SKIN

Carrot Seed	Clary Sage	Sandalwood
Marjoram	Lavender	Neroli
Roman Chamomile	Orange	Mandarin
Geranium	Palmarosa	Jasmine
Rose	Rosewood	Spikenard
Myrrh	Petitgrain	Patchouli
Cedarwood	Ylang Ylang	Helichrysum

OILY SKIN

Bergamot	Juniper	Geranium
Mandarin	Lemongrass	Clary Sage
Tea Tree	Basil	Cedarwood
Grapefruit	Niaouli	Ylang Ylang
Lemon	Lavender	Peppermint
Nutmeg	Cypress	Cajeput

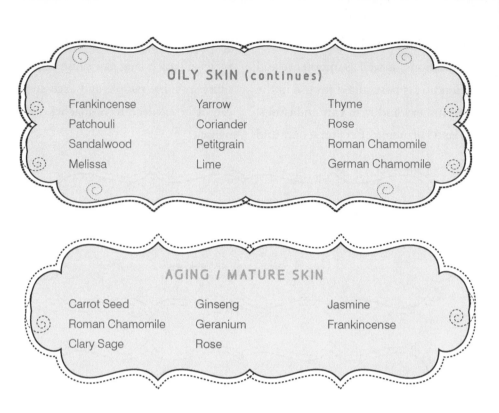

OILY SKIN (continues)

Frankincense	Yarrow	Thyme
Patchouli	Coriander	Rose
Sandalwood	Petitgrain	Roman Chamomile
Melissa	Lime	German Chamomile

AGING / MATURE SKIN

Carrot Seed	Ginseng	Jasmine
Roman Chamomile	Geranium	Frankincense
Clary Sage	Rose	

SKIN CARE SPECIAL CONDITIONS

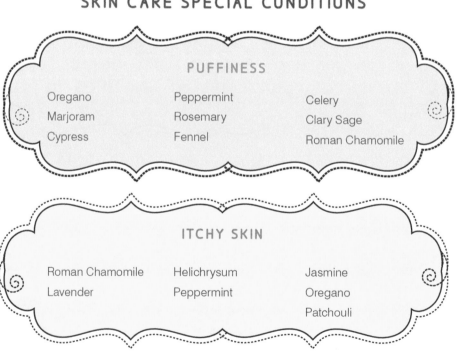

PUFFINESS

Oregano	Peppermint	Celery
Marjoram	Rosemary	Clary Sage
Cypress	Fennel	Roman Chamomile

ITCHY SKIN

Roman Chamomile	Helichrysum	Jasmine
Lavender	Peppermint	Oregano
		Patchouli

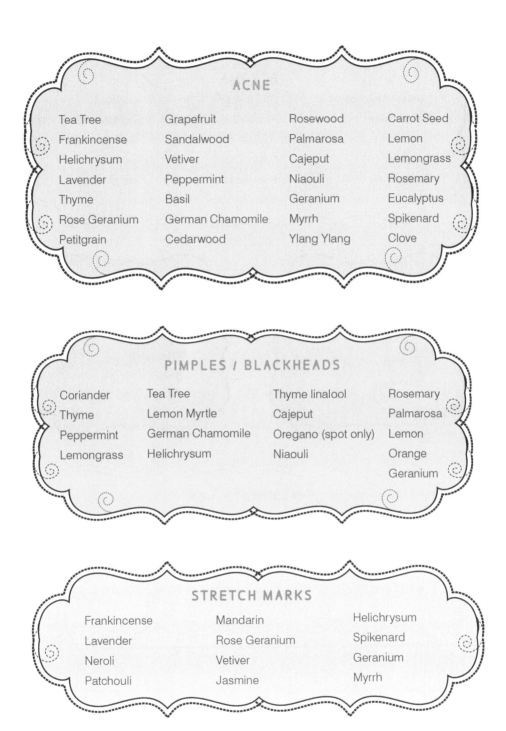

ACNE

Tea Tree	Grapefruit	Rosewood	Carrot Seed
Frankincense	Sandalwood	Palmarosa	Lemon
Helichrysum	Vetiver	Cajeput	Lemongrass
Lavender	Peppermint	Niaouli	Rosemary
Thyme	Basil	Geranium	Eucalyptus
Rose Geranium	German Chamomile	Myrrh	Spikenard
Petitgrain	Cedarwood	Ylang Ylang	Clove

PIMPLES / BLACKHEADS

Coriander	Tea Tree	Thyme linalool	Rosemary
Thyme	Lemon Myrtle	Cajeput	Palmarosa
Peppermint	German Chamomile	Oregano (spot only)	Lemon
Lemongrass	Helichrysum	Niaouli	Orange
			Geranium

STRETCH MARKS

Frankincense	Mandarin	Helichrysum
Lavender	Rose Geranium	Spikenard
Neroli	Vetiver	Geranium
Patchouli	Jasmine	Myrrh

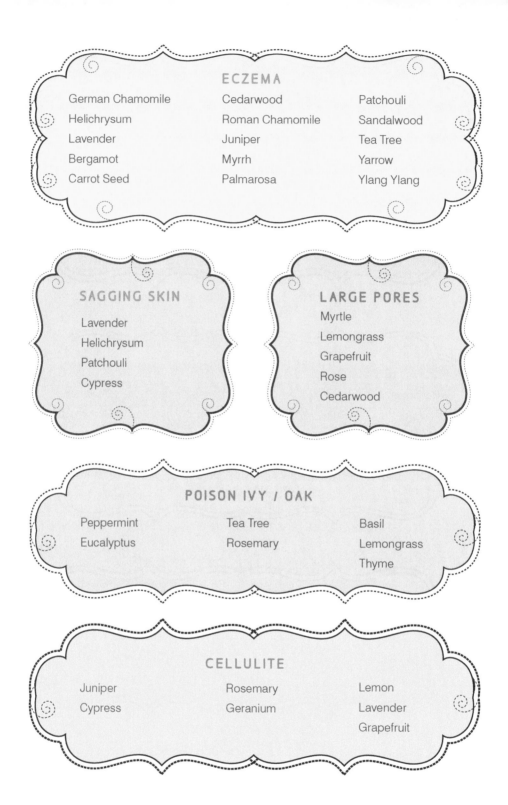

ECZEMA

German Chamomile
Helichrysum
Lavender
Bergamot
Carrot Seed

Cedarwood
Roman Chamomile
Juniper
Myrrh
Palmarosa

Patchouli
Sandalwood
Tea Tree
Yarrow
Ylang Ylang

SAGGING SKIN

Lavender
Helichrysum
Patchouli
Cypress

LARGE PORES

Myrtle
Lemongrass
Grapefruit
Rose
Cedarwood

POISON IVY / OAK

Peppermint
Eucalyptus

Tea Tree
Rosemary

Basil
Lemongrass
Thyme

CELLULITE

Juniper
Cypress

Rosemary
Geranium

Lemon
Lavender
Grapefruit

SCARS

Helichrysum (in a base of Rosehip Seed oil)

Carrot Seed
Lavender

Petitgrain
Galbanum

SENSITIVE SKIN

Roman Chamomile
German Chamomile
Lavender
Rose

Palmarosa
Helichrysum
Neroli
Rosewood

Carrot Seed
Angelica
Jasmine
Sandalwood

SKIN INFECTIONS

German Chamomile
Eucalyptus
Lavender
Myrrh
Roman Chamomile

Rosemary
Spikenard
Tea Tree
Thyme linalool
Calendula
Palmarosa

Niaouli
Myrtle
Rosewood
Oregano
Tea Tree

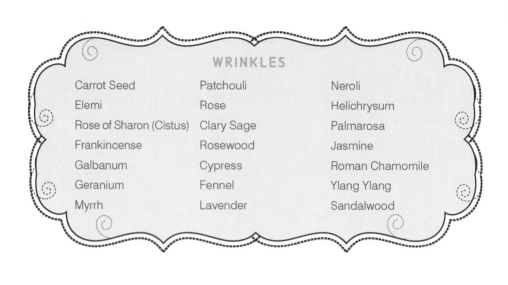

WRINKLES

Carrot Seed	Patchouli	Neroli
Elemi	Rose	Helichrysum
Rose of Sharon (Cistus)	Clary Sage	Palmarosa
Frankincense	Rosewood	Jasmine
Galbanum	Cypress	Roman Chamomile
Geranium	Fennel	Ylang Ylang
Myrrh	Lavender	Sandalwood

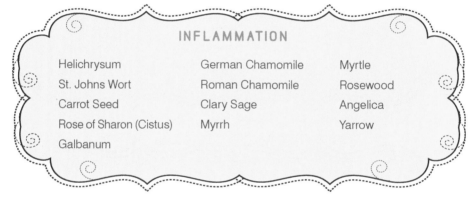

INFLAMMATION

Helichrysum	German Chamomile	Myrtle
St. Johns Wort	Roman Chamomile	Rosewood
Carrot Seed	Clary Sage	Angelica
Rose of Sharon (Cistus)	Myrrh	Yarrow
Galbanum		

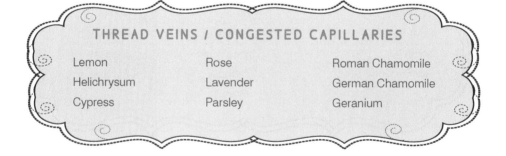

THREAD VEINS / CONGESTED CAPILLARIES

Lemon	Rose	Roman Chamomile
Helichrysum	Lavender	German Chamomile
Cypress	Parsley	Geranium

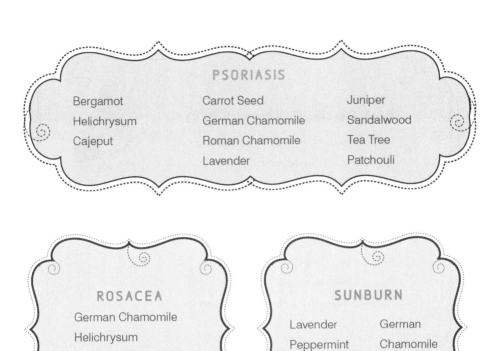

PSORIASIS

Bergamot	Carrot Seed	Juniper
Helichrysum	German Chamomile	Sandalwood
Cajeput	Roman Chamomile	Tea Tree
	Lavender	Patchouli

ROSACEA

German Chamomile
Helichrysum
Rosewood

SUNBURN

Lavender	German
Peppermint	Chamomile
Helichrysum	

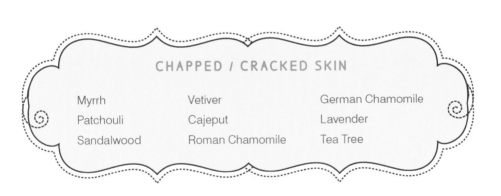

CHAPPED / CRACKED SKIN

Myrrh	Vetiver	German Chamomile
Patchouli	Cajeput	Lavender
Sandalwood	Roman Chamomile	Tea Tree

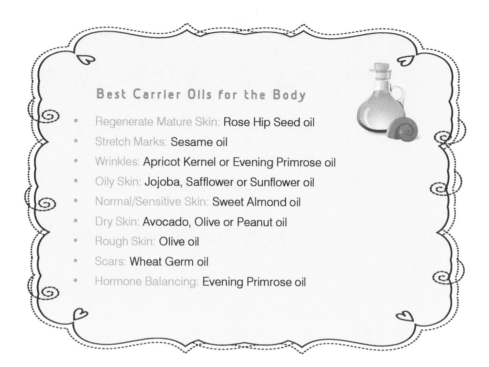

Best Carrier Oils for the Body

- Regenerate Mature Skin: **Rose Hip Seed oil**
- Stretch Marks: **Sesame oil**
- Wrinkles: **Apricot Kernel or Evening Primrose oil**
- Oily Skin: **Jojoba, Safflower or Sunflower oil**
- Normal/Sensitive Skin: **Sweet Almond oil**
- Dry Skin: **Avocado, Olive or Peanut oil**
- Rough Skin: **Olive oil**
- Scars: **Wheat Germ oil**
- Hormone Balancing: **Evening Primrose oil**

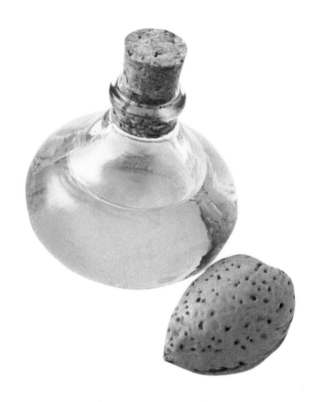

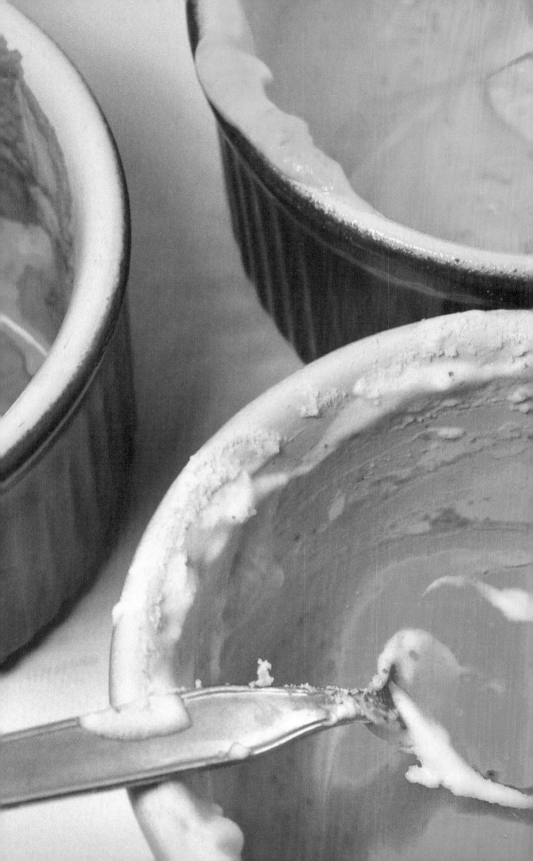

Homemade
Natural Food Coloring

Most commercial bath and body products today contain coloring dyes made from harmful chemicals. This is why making your own homemade skincare products is a good idea. Keeping your own organic bath products free from toxins includes keeping your coloring agents natural, healthy, and allergen free. Follow these simple recipes below to create easy and safe botanically-based food coloring using fruits and vegetables from your kitchen. These will keep up to two weeks when stored in the refrigerator. Simply add several drops when color is desired or called for in a bath recipe.

JOLLY GREEN FOOD COLORING

What You Will Need:

2 cups Spinach leaves (or any green fruit or vegetable)

Water

Pot

Glass container

What To Do:

1. And spinach leaves to a pot. Cover with cold water.
2. Boil for 1 minute then turn heat setting to low and simmer for 10 minutes.
3. Remove from heat and let cool. Strain liquid through fine cheesecloth or wire strainer.
4. Store liquid in a glass container with lid.

BERRY BLUE FOOD COLORING

What You Will Need:

1 cup Blueberries (or any purple/blue fruit or vegetable)

1-2 cups Water

Pot

Glass container

What to Do:

1. Add the blueberries (fresh or frozen) and water to a pot.
2. Simmer on the stove for 20-30 minutes.
3. Leave in pan to cool for 15 minutes. Pour mixture into a blender and pulverize for 1 minute.
4. Pour liquid through a cheesecloth or a mesh strainer into a glass container. Cover with lid and store in the refrigerator until ready to use.

RUBY RED FOOD COLORING

What You Will Need:

2-3 Beets (or any red fruit or vegetable)

2 teaspoons White Vinegar

Water

Pot

Glass container

What To Do:

1. Add the beets (unpeeled is fine) to a pot. Cover with water.

2. Simmer for 45 minutes or until tender.

3. Leave in pan until cool. Remove the beets. Peel, slice and chop them, reserving the juice. Return chopped beets to the pan of water.

4. Let the beets sit in the pan for several hours so the water can absorb the red coloring from the beets.

5. Strain the liquid through a fine cheesecloth or wire strainer. Add vinegar and stir.

6. Pour red mixture to a clean glass container with lid. Store in the refrigerator until ready to use.

Recipe Variation: Other red fruits or vegetables you can use to create your red food coloring include: cranberries, strawberries, rhubarb, tomatoes, red onions or pomegranates. If using cranberries, cover with water and boil for two hours. Mash cranberries until they soften then strain liquid.

MELLOW YELLOW FOOD COLORING

What You Will Need:

1 tablespoon Turmeric (or any yellow fruit or vegetable)

1 cup Water

Pot

Glass container

What To Do:

1. Bring water to a boil. Remove from heat and let cool for 1 minute.

2. Add the turmeric to the water and stir. Continue to add more turmeric until it reaches the intensity you desire.

3. Strain the liquid mixture through a cheesecloth or wire strainer into a glass container. Store in container with tight lid in the refrigerator until ready to use.

Recipe Variation: Other yellow fruits and vegetables you can use to create your yellow food coloring include: curry, squash, yellow beets, outer skins of yellow onions, saffron, daffodil, acacia, or crocus blossoms and carrots. For onion skins, boil for 10 minutes until dark yellow then strain. For flower blossoms, boil for 1 minute then simmer for 2 hours, until it reaches the desired color. For brown food coloring, use cocoa, tea bags or coffee beans.

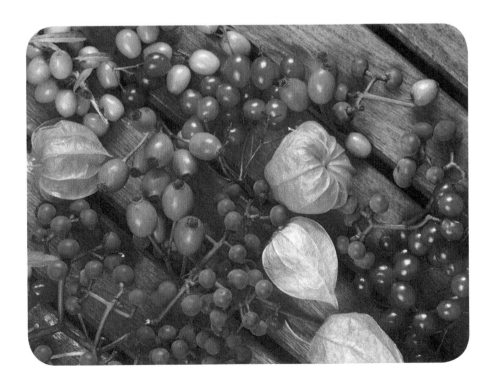

Natural Food Coloring Tips

- Do not store your food coloring in plastic containers as plastic will stain and chemicals in the plastic will contaminate the liquid.

- Try experimenting with different herbs and vegetables to create your food coloring.

- To intensify color, add additional fruit or vegetables to the water and let sit until the solution has reached the shade you want. Remove when you have the desired consistency and shade.

- Natural food coloring can be stored in the refrigerator up to 2 weeks.

- Be careful working with plant materials that you are unfamiliar with. Make sure small children or pets don't eat or drink the materials.

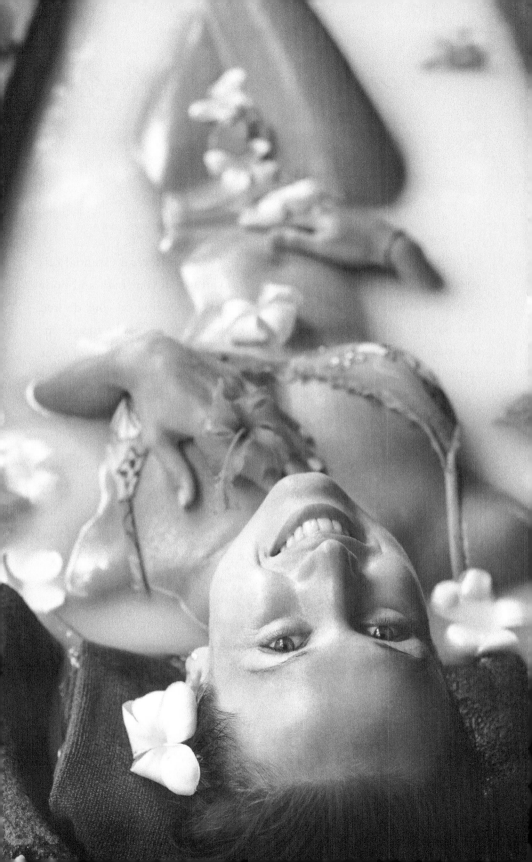

Essential Care for the Body

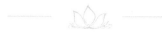

Looking for that perfect all-natural bath product? One that will keep your skin looking great, is appealing to smell, has actual therapeutic benefits without all the chemicals, and oh, doesn't break the bank? Look no further!

You will find a luxurious array of eco-friendly bath and beauty recipes included in this book that will satisfy you from head to toe. Creating a wonderful shower gel, bubble bath, bath fizzy or bath oil for your skin type with the magic of potent natural botanicals can be a rewarding experience. Drawn from essential oils' well-known skin rejuvenating effects, these formulas are designed with the naturalist in mind. Each recipe is filled with wonderful fragrances and soothing, rich organic ingredients. And, knowing the best essential oil for your skin type helps you bring balance and harmony to your body and spirit.

There are several essential oils you can use in your bath and body recipes, depending on your desired results. Some oils may be added simply to enhance the aroma of your blend; others may be included in your blend for their known benefit such as relieving tension or to bring about a healthy state of mind—most natural clinicians will tell you that beauty starts from the inside-out.

You may be asking, "Does this mean I have to spend more to make organic bath products?" While a few of the most highly regarded therapeutic grade essential oils may seem expensive, they are effective in such small concentration it really makes them worth the cost. You will find though, the majority of aromatic oils affordable that can easily become a part of your regular beauty routine at very little cost to you. And their efficacy is well known; that's why so many laboratory-made preparations use components of essential oils in their formulas.

Now you too, can make bath and body products you will love that makes your skin glow.

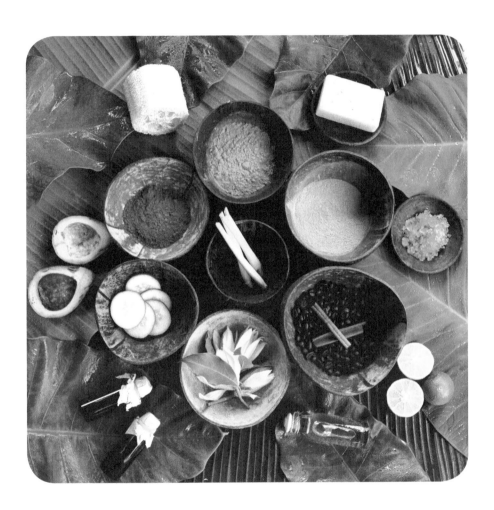

Bath Oils

One of the best ways to keep your skin soft and silky is with bath oils. Why not try one today? Step into a relaxing and luxurious bathing experience and soothe your tiredness and aches away.

It's no wonder bath oils have been used by every culture for thousands of years. As a sensual body ritual, women understood that bath oils not only helped to retain their skin's youthful glow but that they reduced cellulite and fat, promoted healing, and relieved stress.

As an aromatic experience in the shower or bath, you will benefit from the essential oils in your bath oil in a number of ways. Your skin will easily absorb the oils carrying nutrients to those necessary areas via the bloodstream. When used in a hot shower or bath, the fragrant steam is inhaled which stimulates the limbic region (emotional center) of the brain—in-

creasing a sense of well-being.

And, after a hard day at work, there are few things more satisfying than a bath to help reduce aches, pains, or joint stiffness. In addition, aromatic baths are excellent for skin troubles, circulatory problems, respiratory symptoms, stress and nervous tension, insomnia, and menstrual pain. As a bath for detoxifying the body, using the right combination of essential oils can eliminate your body of toxins, helping you lose weight and get healthy.

You can even dress up your oils with interesting colorful bottles and small décor dropped in. Why not give these as gifts to family and friends for the holidays? Personalize them with a label and blend name like "Caroline's Garden Bath Oil" or "Rachel's Romantic Bath Oil." These will show just how special they are to you.

GARDEN BATH OIL

What You Will Need:

4 tablespoons Sweet Almond oil

12 drops Sandalwood essential oil

8 drops Orange essential oil

4 drops Rose essential oil

2 drops Lemon essential oil

Dark glass bottle

What To Do:

1. Mix all of the ingredients together and store in a dark bottle.
2. Add 1 tablespoon of the scented oil to a warm bath and swish the water around. Relax in your bath for at least 15 minutes.

CIRCULATORY BATH OIL

Cypress essential oil is known for alleviating circulatory problems and Orange essential oil helps with dry skin.

What You Will Need:

½ ounce Sweet Almond oil

4 drops Cypress essential oil

4 drops Orange essential oil

What You Will Need:

1. Combine oils and add to a running bath.
2. Soak for 15-20 minutes.

ZEST BATH OIL

Enjoy a relaxing and invigorating bath!

What You Will Need:

3 1/3 ounces Sweet Almond oil

2/3 ounce Wheat Germ oil

25 drops Grapefruit essential oil

25 drops Coriander essential oil

What To Do:

1. Mix all the above ingredients together and store in a dark bottle.
2. Add about 1 tablespoon of your scented oil to a warm bath and swish the water around. Relax and enjoy your bath for at least 15 minutes.

TONING OIL

Use this oil before taking a bath or shower!

What You Will Need:

4 drops Black Pepper essential oil

3 drops Ginger essential oil

1 drop Parsley essential oil

6 drops Lemongrass essential oil

What To Do:

1. In a bottle or small jar, combine the essential oils and shake to blend well.
2. Use 5 drops of the toning oil with 1 teaspoon of Sweet Almond oil or another carrier oil.
3. Massage all over body before getting into the bath or shower.

MILK & HONEY BATH OIL

What You Will Need:

1 cup Honey

2 cups Milk

1 cup Salt

¼ cup Baking Soda

½ cup Jojoba oil

Essential oil (your choice)

Bowl

What To Do:

1. In a bowl, combine the honey, milk, and salt.
2. Add the Jojoba oil and a few drops of the essential oil.
3. Fill your tub and pour the mixture in.

LEMON TWIST BATH OIL

What You Will Need:

¼ cup Sweet Almond oil

¼ cup Vinegar

¼ teaspoon Lemon essential oil

¼ teaspoon Bergamot essential oil

2 teaspoons Lemon juice

What To Do:

1. Place all of the ingredients in a sealable glass container or jar.
2. Replace lid and shake well. This one will create a very interesting effect as the oils and the vinegar will keep separating from one another. Just remember before using to give it another good shake.

GERANIUM & OLIVE BATH OIL

What You Will Need:

3 tablespoons Olive oil

8 drops Geranium essential oil

What To Do:

1. Combine the olive oil and essential oil and pour into a running bath.
2. Soak for 15 minutes.

ORANGE & SPEARMINT BATH OIL

This is a mind-easing blend for total relaxation.

What You Will Need:

½ cup Coconut oil

½ teaspoon Spearmint essential oil

½ teaspoon Orange essential oil

Bottle

What To Do:

1. Simply add all three ingredients together in a bottle or a jar. Shake well.
2. Add to a running bath and soak.

ARTHRITIS RELIEF BATH OIL

What You Will Need:

1 cup Sweet Almond oil

15 drops Lavender essential oil

8 drops Clary Sage essential oil

7 drops Ylang Ylang essential oil

Bottle

What To Do:

1. Combine the essential oils and almond oil in a bottle.
2. Shake well to mix then add a couple of tablespoons to running water.
3. Soak for 15 minutes.

BACKACHE RELIEF BATH OIL

Thyme essential oil, well known for its medicinal properties, works together with Eucalyptus to help relieve back and joint pain.

What You Will Need:

1 cup Sweet Almond oil

15 drops Thyme essential oil

5 drops Eucalyptus essential oil

Bottle

What To Do:

1. Combine the essential oils and almond oil in a bottle or jar.
2. Shake well to mix then add a couple of tablespoons to running water.
3. Soak for 15 minutes.

HAWAIIAN BATH OIL

Enjoy the wonderful tropical aroma as your body soaks up the oils.

What You Will Need:

1/8 cup Canola oil

1/8 cup Apricot oil

10 drops Mango oil

10 drops Coconut oil

10 drops Gardenia essential oil

Bottle

What To Do:

1. Mix all of the ingredients thoroughly together in a bottle until ready for use.
2. When ready, add to the warm running water as you fill your bathtub and then soak.

PMS BATH OIL

Relax and soak yourself while the oils do the work.

What You Will Need:

1/8 cup Sweet Almond oil

1/8 cup Grapeseed oil

3 drops Clary Sage oil

3 drops Lavender essential oil

2 drops Rose absolute oil

2 drops Juniper essential oil

Bottle

What To Do:

1. Add all of the oils together in a bottle and shake well.
2. To use, add the oils to your warm running bath water and mix well. Relax and soak for 15-20 minutes. If your stomach and abdomen are bloated, you can use a few drops of the oils to rub gently and directly onto the area.

ROMANCE BATH OIL

Allow your senses to stimulate your thoughts as well as warm your body, mind, and soul.

What You Will Need:

4 drops Ylang Ylang essential oil

4 drops Frankincense essential oil

4 drops Jasmine essential oil

4 drops Sandalwood essential oil

4 drops Rose essential oil

What To Do:

1. Measure out the ingredients as needed above, drop by drop, placing them under the flow of your warm running bath water.

2. Add a lit candle or two and take time out to relax and enjoy yourself.

SWEET 'N SOFT BATH OIL

Enjoy the warm wonderful aroma of a bath as your body soaks up the oils.

What You Will Need:

1/8 cup Soybean oil

1/8 cup Jojoba oil

½ teaspoon Honey

15 drops Rosemary essential oil

12 drops Lemon essential oil

5 drops Sandalwood essential oil

Bottle

What To Do:

1. Add all of the ingredients together in a bottle and shake well to blend.

2. Pour a few tablespoons into warm running water as you fill your bathtub.

RELAXING LAVENDER HONEY BATH OIL

Did you know that honey has a calming effect? Combined with the pure essential oil of Lavender, it's a yummy bath treatment. Why not try it tonight!

What You Will Need:

2 ounces Honey

5 drops Lavender essential oil

What To Do:

1. Combine the honey and Lavender in a jar. Shake well.

2. Use 1-2 tablespoons per bath.

VARICOSE VEINS BATH OIL

This bath includes essential oils that can help boost circulation in the legs such as Ginger, Juniper, Lemon, Rosemary, and Cypress.

What You Will Need:

2 drops Ginger essential oil

2 drops Rosemary essential oil

2 drops Lemon essential oil

4 drops Juniper essential oil

4 drops Cypress essential oil

1 ounce Sweet Almond oil

Bottle or jar

What To Do:

1.   In a bottle or jar, add essential oils and Sweet Almond oil. Blend well.

2.   Add to a bath of warm running water.

FLU BUSTER BATH OIL

What You Will Need:

2 drops Cinnamon essential oil

2 drops Lemon essential oil

2 drops Clove essential oil

2 drops Rosemary essential oil

2 drops Tea Tree essential oil

2 drops Eucalyptus essential oil

1 ounce Sweet Almond oil

Small, dark glass

bottle

What To Do:

1.   In a small dark bottle, add all of the oils and shake to blend well.

2.   Add in a very warm bath, swishing around to distribute.

MEDITATION BATH OIL

What You Will Need:

½ ounce Sweet Almond oil

5 drops Sandalwood essential oil

5 drops Rose essential oil

5 drops Lavender essential oil

½ teaspoon Mandarin essential oil

Small dark glass

bottle

What To Do:

1. Combine all of the ingredients in a small dark glass bottle. Shake to mix thoroughly.

2. Add to running bath water. As you soak, meditate upon a favorite verse or saying.

LEMONGRASS SKIN CONDITIONER

This conditioner works well for oily and scaly skin.

What You Will Need:

1 quart Distilled Water

1 ounce Lemongrass essential oil

1 ounce Cornmeal

1 ounce Witch Hazel

1 ounce Rose petals

What To Do:

1. In a bowl, add Lemongrass essential oil, cornmeal, witch hazel and rose petals.

2. Pour this mixture into a quart of boiling water.

3. Let steep 20 minutes. Strain liquid.

4. Add 1 ounce of liquid to bath water. Soak at least 10 minutes.

5. Use twice a week.

FOAMING BATH OIL BALLS

What You Will Need:

¼ cup Baking Soda

2 tablespoons Citric acid or Ascorbic acid

1 tablespoon Borax Powder (for softening)

2 tablespoons Powdered Sugar (for binding)

2 tablespoons Sweet Almond oil

1 teaspoon Vitamin E oil (preservative)

¼ teaspoon essential oil (your choice)

What To Do:

1. Combine the dry ingredients in a bowl and stir until well blended.
2. Drizzle in almond oil and stir until mixture is moistened.
3. Add vitamin E oil and fragrance, and stir until well mixed.
4. Take teaspoon-sized globs of mixture and form into balls. If the mixture is too crumbly and won't hold together, add a little more vitamin E oil.
5. Place the balls on a sheet of wax paper and set on the counter for 2-3 hours.
6. When time is up, reshape balls. Let them air-dry and harden for ten days.
7. Store balls in a closed container to protect from moisture.
8. To use, plop a ball into your bathtub in warm water!

CUSTOM-SCENTED BATH OIL

What You Will Need:

Sunflower oil

Essential oil (your choice)

Corked container

Crystal beads, dried flowers, small seashells, etc. (optional)

What To Do:

1. Pour oil through a funnel into the corked container, leaving about an inch at the top.
2. Add 4 teaspoons of the essential oil per ½ quart.

3. Cork the container and agitate the bottle gently.

4. Let it sit for 2-3 days before using.

5. Add décor to your bottle.

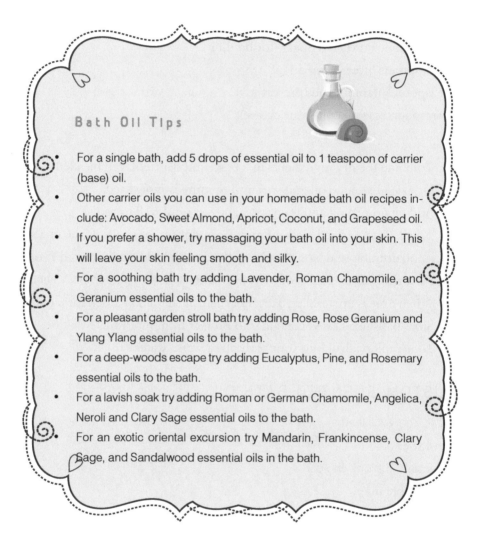

Bath Oil Tips

- For a single bath, add 5 drops of essential oil to 1 teaspoon of carrier (base) oil.
- Other carrier oils you can use in your homemade bath oil recipes include: Avocado, Sweet Almond, Apricot, Coconut, and Grapeseed oil.
- If you prefer a shower, try massaging your bath oil into your skin. This will leave your skin feeling smooth and silky.
- For a soothing bath try adding Lavender, Roman Chamomile, and Geranium essential oils to the bath.
- For a pleasant garden stroll bath try adding Rose, Rose Geranium and Ylang Ylang essential oils to the bath.
- For a deep-woods escape try adding Eucalyptus, Pine, and Rosemary essential oils to the bath.
- For a lavish soak try adding Roman or German Chamomile, Angelica, Neroli and Clary Sage essential oils to the bath.
- For an exotic oriental excursion try Mandarin, Frankincense, Clary Sage, and Sandalwood essential oils in the bath.

Bath Bombs

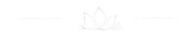

One soap-maker described bath bombs as giant Alka-Seltzers for your bath—they spin, whirl, and swirl in your tub while releasing their scent and skin-softening agents. Even if you're an adult, bath time can still be fun!

These rounded masses begin to fizzle, bubble, and dissolve, usually in a minute or so, when placed in water. You may even hear a hissing or crackling sound as they react with the water. This is because they are usually made of baking soda, Citric acid, cornstarch, or Epsom salt. You can add dried flowers or herbs to your bath bombs that will float along the surface once released. Most bath bomb recipes call for a fragrant oil to further enhance your bathing experience.

Essential oils not only add magnificent fragrance, but also therapeutic benefits. Lavender or Roman Chamomile essential oil, for instance, helps bathers to relax and let go of stress, while adding Sweet Almond oil or Sunflower oil helps to moisturize the skin. Other essential oils such as Rose or Geranium may be added that rejuvenate the skin, leaving it soft.

Bath bombs certainly do make bath time a special occasion, and kids especially love how they crackle and twirl around when they plunk them in the tub! Why not make a few as gifts for friends who might need a little extra pampering?

WILD CITRUS GARDEN BATH KISSES

What You Will Need:

2 ounces Cocoa Butter

2 ounces Baking Soda

2 ounces Citric Acid

3 tablespoons Oatmeal, powdered

10 drops Natural Food Coloring (optional)

10 drops Bergamot essential oil

5 drops Rose essential oil

10 drops Ylang Ylang essential oil

Soap mold

What To Do:

1. Melt the cocoa butter in a microwave or stovetop.
2. Add the food coloring and essential oils. Mix well.
3. Add the baking soda, citric acid and powdered oatmeal. Stir thoroughly.
4. Pour into molds. Place in the freezer to set. This will take about 10-20 minutes.
5. Remove from molds when set. To use, place 1-2 in a running bath; use 3-4 for extra moisturizing.

MRS. SANDMAN'S BATH COOKIES

These are wonderful as gifts, but not as food! For use in the bath only—do not eat.

What You Will Need:

2 cups Sea Salt

½ cup Baking Soda

½ cup Cornstarch

2 tablespoons Sweet Almond oil

1 teaspoon Vitamin E oil

1-2 Eggs

6 drops Lavender essential oil

4 drops Roman Chamomile essential oil

3 drops Natural Yellow Food Coloring (optional)

What To Do:

1. Preheat oven to 350 degrees.
2. Mix all of the ingredients in a bowl together.
3. Shape mixture together by rolling a teaspoon of dough into 1-inch balls or roll out then cut with cookie cutters in the shape you want. (You can decorate the cookies with clove buds, anise seeds, or dried citrus peel if you wish.)
4. Bake the cookies for 10-12 minutes, until lightly browned. Do not over-bake.
5. Allow the cookies to cool completely. To use, drop 1-2 cookies into a warm bath. Store bath cookies in an airtight container. These are perishable because of the eggs so use them up or give as gifts. Yield: 24 cookies or enough for twelve baths.

ENERGY-BOOSTING BATH BOMBS

What You Will Need:

2 tablespoons Citric Acid

2 tablespoons Cornstarch

¼ cup Baking Soda

3 tablespoons Coconut oil (or Sweet Almond, Avocado or Apricot Kernel)

8 drops Orange essential oil

4 drops Ginger essential oil

3-6 drops Natural Food Coloring (optional)

Paper candy cups

What To Do:

1. Place all of the dry ingredients into a bowl and mix well.
2. Place coconut oil into a small glass bowl and add essential oil and food coloring.
3. Slowly add the oil mixture into dry ingredients and mix well.

4. Scoop up small amounts of the mixture and shape into 1-inch balls. Let the balls rest on a sheet of waxed paper for about 2-3 hours, then place each ball into a candy cup to let dry and harden for 24 to 48 hours.

5. Store bombs in a closed, airtight container. To use, drop 1-3 bombs into warm bath water.

SENSUAL JASMINE BATH BOMBS

Jasmine bath bombs are as gorgeous as the plant itself. Dark green leaves surround small, white star-shaped flowers, which when picked at night have wonderful intense aromas. The therapeutic properties of Jasmine oil include: anti-depressant, aphrodisiac, anti-spasmodic, antiseptic, stimulant, and emollient. If you are pregnant, however, you should avoid making Jasmine bath bombs.

What You Will Need:

3 tablespoons Baking Soda

1 tablespoon Citric Acid

5 drops Jasmine essential oil

3 drops Vanilla essential oil

5-10 drops Natural Green Food Coloring

Witch hazel

Bowl

Molds

What To Do:

1. Sieve the baking soda and citric acid and mix in a bowl.

2. Add the food coloring and essential oils slowly.

3. Spritz lightly with witch hazel. Mix together until the mixture doesn't crumble when squeezed.

4. Press into molds. The bath bombs should be taken out of the mold almost immediately and placed on wax paper to dry for at least 48 hours.

MUFFIN TIN VICKS SHOWER DISKS

Feeling stuffy? Place one of these shower disks on the shower floor and let the essential oils and steam help you breathe freely!

What You Will Need:

2-3 cups Baking Soda

15 drops Eucalyptus essential oil

15 drops Lavender essential oil

15 drops Rosemary essential oil

Muffin Tin

Baking Cup Liners

Water

What To Do:

1. In a bowl, add baking soda and a little water at a time until mixture becomes a thick paste.
2. Add essential oils to the mixture.
3. Spoon the mixture into baking cup liners. Allow to sit for 12-16 hours.
4. To use, pop out and place shower muffin on the shower floor when needed.

FIZZY BATH CRYSTALS

What You Will Need:

8 ounces Cornstarch

8 ounces Citric Acid

16 ounces Baking Soda

½ teaspoon Essential oil (your choice)

Jar or container with lid

What To Do:

1. In a bowl, mix the cornstarch and citric acid together thoroughly.
2. Add essential oils as desired. Blend in the baking soda.
3. Store in a container with lid. Use ¼ to ½ cup per bath.

CUSTOM-SCENTED BATH BOMBS

What You Will Need:

1 cup Baking Soda

½ cup Cornstarch

½ cup Citric Acid

15 drops Essential oil (your choice)

10 drops Natural Food Coloring (your choice)

Soap molds

What To Do:

1. Mix all of the ingredients except the food coloring in a bowl.
2. Add the natural food coloring to a small amount of the mix in a separate bowl.
3. Add colored mix to remaining mix and blend.
4. Mist the mixture with a mister so that it holds together but not enough to start fizzing.
5. Pack the mixture into a soap mold. Flip over onto a piece of waxed paper and allow molded fizzy to dry overnight.

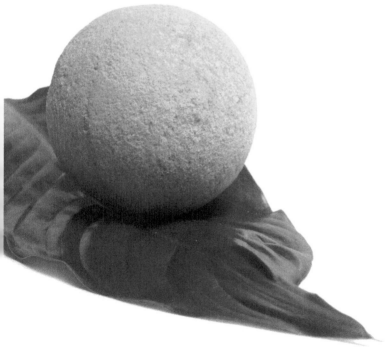

Bath Bomb Tips

- Be careful when choosing a citric acid One that is too fine won't form well; one that is too coarse may leave you with a lumpy appearance.
- For smoother bath bombs, use 10-15% cornstarch as part of your dry ingredient content. This will help with the fizzing action.
- When adding coloring, use cosmetic grade colorant or natural food coloring from a health food store. Or, make your own using the recipes found in the chapter, Homemade Natural Food Coloring.
- Always use therapeutic grade essential oils that are safe for use in the bath.
- Don't use water for binding your mixture because this will cause fizzing and expansion in the mixing process. Instead, add vegetable carrier oils such as Sweet Almond or Grapeseed—witch hazel also works well. Witch hazel will also speed the drying time so that your bath bombs can be safely handled and removed from their molds within minutes.
- Spray your wet ingredients onto the mixture. If using witch hazel to bind, always spritz from a fine mist spray bottle. Oil can be "dripped" or sprayed into your mix. Spraying helps distribute the oil more evenly with less risk of fizzing in the bowl.
- Wear gloves and mix with your hands. Simply spray or pour with one hand while mixing with the other.
- Make sure your molds are completely dry. If the mold gets wet, the bath bomb may get stuck in the mold and refuse to come out. If this happens, run the whole mold under the tap to remove (instead of breaking the mold). Otherwise, you can take the bath bomb mold and all into the bath with you!
- Try not to over-wet your mixture. Make it damp enough to hold together, like wet sand for building a sandcastle, but not sloppy and formless. If mixture does become over-wet, add more dry ingredients.
- Use a melon ball tool to form your bath bombs. Set them onto wax paper to dry. Allow them to set at least one day (or longer), depending on the time of year, temperature, and humidity.
- Work in a cool, dry place. Keep your bath bombs away from water or moisture.

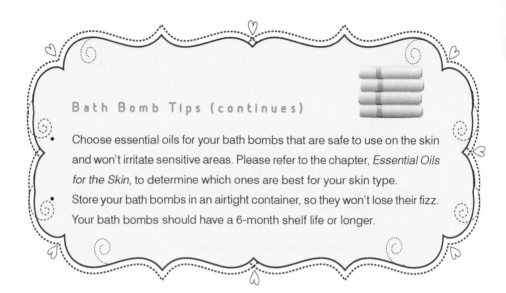

Bath Bomb Tips (continues)

- Choose essential oils for your bath bombs that are safe to use on the skin and won't irritate sensitive areas. Please refer to the chapter, *Essential Oils for the Skin*, to determine which ones are best for your skin type.
- Store your bath bombs in an airtight container, so they won't lose their fizz. Your bath bombs should have a 6-month shelf life or longer.

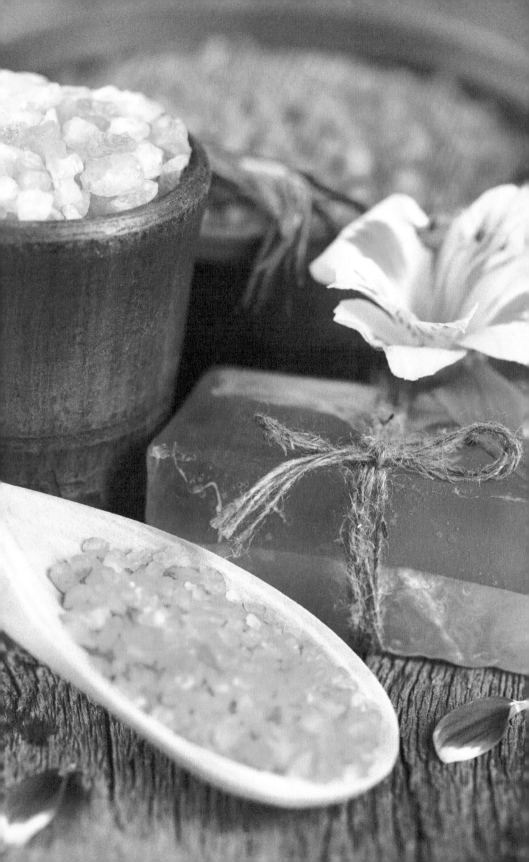

Bath Salts

Aromatic baths are a wonderful natural alternative to modern medicine when it comes to treating common ailments and mood swings. You will find many types of sea salt beauty products on the market today that can easily be made at home.

Salts for the bath alone have many therapeutic properties. The most popular areas salts come from include the Himalayas, the Dead Sea, the Pacific Ocean, the Mediterranean Sea and the Great Salt Lake in Utah, USA. Each kind plays a particular role in the health of our body and skin.

Epsom salt is commonly used as a bath salt and has many benefits such as reducing the prune look of skin. Because the salt changes the osmotic balance of the bath water, it allows your skin to absorb more water.

Magnesium sulphate, one of the main components in bath salts, has anti-inflammatory properties which help the body to stay healthy by avoiding cellular breakdown. Phophates, which are also found in bath salts, soften the skin and calluses, helping to exfoliate the skin and keep it smooth.

Diseases such as a psoriasis and atopic dermatitis are actually treated with high concentrations of sea salt in water; this is why many people with these and other skin ailments go to the Dead Sea for therapy.

Other physical benefits from sea salts include the stimulation of natural circulation, relief from athlete's foot, removing corns and calluses, and relaxation of tense and aching muscles. Rheumatism and arthritis, as well as chronic lower back pain, can be cured with high concentrations of sea salt in water.

Certainly a good sea salt soak can encourage deep relaxation, relief from stress, and will promote restfulness. Sea salt should be one of the main ingredients to have in your bathroom to help you keep your skin and body healthy.

Adding essential oils to your sea salt will benefit you in two ways: through the connection of your olfactory sense with the molecules carried by the steam of the hot bath, and by absorption through the skin. Aromatic bath salts work wonders for the body and are excellent for skin problems, circulatory issues, respiratory problems, stress and nervous tension, muscular aches and pains, and insomnia. The bath salts help to disperse essential oils safely into the water, especially when a carrier oil such as Sweet Almond or Jojoba is added. Without salts or an emulsifier, the drops of essential oils end up floating on top of the water and come in direct contact with the skin.

Below you will find wonderful aromatherapy recipes for adding to a tub of warm water for a relaxing and/ or invigorating bath.

TRANQUIL BATH SALTS

Choose from these oils for a tranquil bath: Cedarwood, Roman Chamomile, Cypress, Frankincense, Geranium, Lavender, Mandarin, Marjoram, Melissa, Myrtle, Neroli, Orange, Petitgrain, Rose, Rosewood, Sandalwood, Valerian, Vanilla, Vetiver, and Ylang Ylang.

What You Will Need:

3 tablespoons Sea Salt, or

2 tablespoons Epsom Salt and 1 tablespoon Sea Salt, or

1 tablespoon Powdered Red Earth Clay and 2 tablespoons Sea Salt, or

1 tablespoon Powdered Kelp and 2 tablespoons Sea Salt

3 tablespoons Baking Soda

8 drops Essential oil (your choice)

4-ounce jar

What To Do:

1. Choose a carrier salt.
2. Choose 3-4 oils from the list above.

3. Add salts, baking soda and essential oils to a jar. If you want your salts to fizz, add 1 tablespoon citric acid. Gently shake to mix well.

   To use, add to a tub of running water.

SALT GLOW

What You Will Need:

¼ cup Sweet Almond oil

¼ cup Melt and Pour Glycerin soap

½ cup Sea Salt

10-12 drops Essential oil (your choice)

Natural Food Coloring (optional)

Wide-mouth jar

What To Do:

1. Place oil and soap in double boiler and melt slowly. Stir well.
2. Slowly stir in sea salt, and remove from heat.
3. Add fragrance of choice and natural food coloring if you like.
4. Add a label to give as a gift. You may want to add instructions to stir well if the ingredients separate. It is very thick.

TANGERINE DREAM BATH SALTS

What You Will Need:

2 drops Roman Chamomile essential oil

7 drops Lavender essential oil

9 drops Tangerine essential oil

3 tablespoons Sea Salt

2 tablespoons Baking Soda

1 tablespoon Borax Powder

What To Do:

1. Add sea salt, baking soda, borax and oils to a jar.
2. Gently shake to mix well.
3. To use, add to a tub of running water.

TOXIN ELIMINATOR BATH

What You Will Need:

2 handfuls Epsom salt

1 handful Sea Salt

8 drops Basil essential oil

10 drops Grapefruit essential oil

6 drops Juniper essential oil

10 drops Lemon essential oil

6 drops Oregano essential oil

Dark glass bottle

What To Do:

1. In a small, dark glass bottle, add the essential oils and shake to blend.
2. Add salts and 8 drops of the blend to a running bath.
3. Massage the cellulite areas while they are under the water.

COUNTRY GARDEN BATH SALTS

What You Will Need:

1 cup Sea Salt

1 cup Epsom Salt

1 cup Baking Soda

6 drops Lavender essential oil

6 drops Rose Geranium essential oil

6 drops Ylang Ylang essential oil

6 drops Helichrysum essential oil

Jar or container

What To Do:

1. In a large container or bowl, mix the salts and baking soda.
2. Stir in each essential oil slowly. Store in a container with a lid. You'll want about 6 drops of essential oils per ¼ cup salt blend.
3. To use, add ¼ cup into a bath of running water.

GLISTENING WINTER NIGHTS BATH SALTS

This bath salts recipe will calm any holiday stress on a winter's night. Plus, you will love the glittery sheen.

What You Will Need:

1 cup Epsom Salt

1 cup Baking Soda

10 drops Natural Blue Food Coloring

¼ cup Fine Silver Glitter

15 drops Lavender essential oil

10 drops Sandalwood essential oil

10 drops Orange essential oil

2 Jars or containers with lids

What To Do:

1. In a large bowl, mix together salts and baking soda.
2. Add the essential oils, mixing well.
3. Add coloring, starting with 8 drops. Add more, until you are pleased with the color. Mix well.
4. Stir in glitter.
5. To use in the bath, add ¼ cup of bath salts to running water.

PICK ME UP BATH SALTS

What You Will Need:

1 cup Epsom Salt

1 tablespoon Baking Soda

1 cup Sea Salt (or substitute 2 cups Epsom Salt)

4 drops Peppermint essential oil

3 drops Rosemary essential oil

3 drops Ginger or Nutmeg essential oil

Natural Food Coloring (optional)

What To Do:

1. Mix salts and baking soda together.

2. Add food coloring to the mixture of salts. Stir in the essential oils slowly. Mix well.

3. Let sit covered for a few hours. Pour into a pretty bottle and tag for gift giving.

ZESTY ROSEMARY BATH SALTS

What You Will Need:

3 cups Sea Salt

3 tablespoons Baking Soda

1 drop Natural Red Food Coloring

1 drop Natural Yellow Food Coloring

5 drops Lemon essential oil

5 drops Rosemary essential oil

Jar

What To Do:

1. In a bowl, mix together all of the ingredients.

2. Stir well. Pour into a jar with a lid.

3. To use, add ¼ cup to running bath water.

DETOX BATH SALTS

What You Will Need:

2 handfuls Epsom Salt

2 handfuls Sea Salt

1 ounce Sweet Almond oil

4 drops Rosemary essential oil

4 drops Violet Leaf essential oil

Container

What To Do:

1. In a large container, mix salts.

2. In another bowl, mix carrier oil and essential oils. Stir well.

3. Add essential oil blend to salts and mix well.

4. To use, add ¼ cup to a running bath.

ORANGE & TANGERINE BATH SOAK

What You Will Need:

½ cup Baking Soda

¼ cup Epsom Salt

¼ teaspoon Orange essential oil

¼ teaspoon Tangerine essential oil

1 drop Natural Red Food Coloring

1 drop Natural Yellow Food Coloring

What To Do:

1. Combine the salts and baking soda.
2. Stir in food coloring and essential oils until evenly distributed.
3. Transfer mixture into a food processor and grind into a fine powder.
4. Spoon into a jar. To use, add ¼ cup to a running bath.

PEACH HARVEST BATH SALTS

What You Will Need:

3 cups Epsom Salt

1 cup Sea Salt

½ cup Baking Soda

10 drops Peach essential oil

10 drops Bergamot essential oil

7 drops Vanilla essential oil

3 drops Orange essential oil

1-2 drops Natural Red Food Coloring

1-2 drops Natural Yellow Food Coloring

Jar with lid

What To Do:

1. Mix the salts and baking soda together.
2. In a small bowl, combine the oils and add the food coloring. Stir well.

3. Add the oil/coloring to the salt mixture and stir well. Let stand allowing the color and scent to penetrate through.
4. To use, add ½ to 1 cup in a bath of running water.

OCEAN BLUE BATH SALTS

What You Will Need:

1 cup Epsom Salt

1 cup Baking Soda

4 drops Natural Blue Food Coloring

3 drops Jasmine essential oil

4 drops Vanilla essential oil

2 tablespoons Glycerin

What To Do:

1. Combine all of dry ingredients and mix well.
2. Add color and essential oils one at a time. Break up any clumps and keep mixing until you have a semi-fine powder.
3. Add glycerin and mix well.
4. To use, add ½ to 1 cup in a bath of running water.

SPRING AWAKENINGS BATH SALTS

What You Will Need:

1 cup Epsom Salt

1 cup Baking Soda

3 drops Natural Red Food Coloring

3 drops Natural Yellow Food Coloring

10 drops Orange essential oil

15 drops Ylang Ylang essential oil

What To Do:

1. In a large bowl, mix together the salts and baking soda.
2. Add essential oils, mixing well.

3. Add the food coloring, starting with 2 drops of red and 3 of yellow. Mix well. Add another drop of red if needed—you are going for a peach color. This recipe makes 2 cups.
4. To use, add 4 tablespoons of bath salts to running water for one full tub.

ASPEN DREAMS BATH SALTS

This fragrant bath will remind you of the great outdoors with its woodsy scent and is great for soothing achy muscles after a hike. It offers a very masculine tone, but women will love it too!

What You Will Need:

2 cups Epsom Salt

2 tablespoons Baking Soda

5 drops Rosewood essential oil

2 drops Cedarwood essential oil

2 drops Roman Chamomile essential oil

1-2 drops Natural Yellow Food Coloring

1-2 drops Natural Red Food Coloring

Jar with lid

What To Do:

1. In a bowl, add the salts and baking soda and mix well.
2. In a separate glass, add the essential oils and food coloring then stir, blending well. Pour them evenly over the salt and stir to mix well.
3. Let sit for over an hour before placing in a jar and sealing.

AUTUMN PEACH BATH SALTS

This bath salt recipe helps de-stress you with its soothing autumn scent.

What You Will Need:

1 cup Epsom Salt

1 cup Baking Soda

4 drops Natural Red Food Coloring

8 drops Natural Yellow Food Coloring

20 drops Ginger or Cardamom essential oil

10 drops Cinnamon essential oil

Jars or containers with lids

What To Do:

1. In a large bowl, mix together the salts and baking soda.
2. Add all of the essential oils, mixing well.
3. Next, add food coloring, starting with 4 drops of red and 8 of yellow. Mix well. Continue adding 1 drop at a time until you are pleased with the color.
4. For the bath: add 4 heaping tablespoons of bath salts to running water for one full tub. This recipe makes 2 cups.

ENERGIZING BATH SALTS

What You Will Need:

2 cup Epsom Salt

1 cup Sea Salt

10 drops Natural Green Food Coloring

5 drops Natural Blue Food Coloring

6 drops Eucalyptus essential oil

10 drops Rosemary essential oil

15 drops Peppermint essential oil

What To Do:

1. In a large bowl, add salts and food coloring.
2. Add the essential oils, one drop at a time and mix well. Let it sit overnight.
3. For the bath: Add 4 heaping tablespoons of bath salts to running water for one full tub.

NORTHERN NIGHTS BATH SALTS

What You Will Need:

1 cup Dead Sea Salt

1 cup Baking Soda

3 drops Balsam Pine essential oil

2 drops Cinnamon essential oil

2 drops Cassia essential oil

2 tablespoons Glycerin

What To Do:

1. Mix salt and baking soda together.
2. Add glycerin and essential oils together then add to the salt mixture. Break up any clumps.
3. To use, add 2-4 tablespoons of bath salts to running water for a full bath.

NOURISHING BATH SALTS

What You Will Need:

3 cups Sea Salt

3 tablespoons Sweet Almond oil

2 teaspoons Apricot Kernel oil

2 teaspoons Avocado oil

¼ cup Baking Soda

20 drops Sandalwood essential oil

20 drops Rosewood essential oil

10 drops Ylang Ylang essential oil

5 drops German Chamomile essential oil

What To Do:

1. Add salts, carrier oils and baking soda to a bowl and stir well.
2. In another bowl, add all of the essential oils and stir. Pour over salt mixture and blend well.
3. To use, add 4 tablespoons to a running warm bath. Enjoy!

NAKED BEE BATH SALTS

What You Will Need:

1 ½ cups Epsom Salt (or Sea Salt)

1/3 cup Honey

2 drops Natural Yellow Food Coloring

3 drops Orange essential oil

What To Do:

1. Place the salts in a bowl. Add honey. Stir mixture until well blended. It will seem a little sticky.
2. In another bowl, mix yellow food coloring and the essential oil.
3. Stir the oil/color mixture into the salts.
4. Cover bowl and let sit for about 30 minutes.
5. Use ¼ cup of recipe for each bath, dropping into hot running water as tub fills.

GENTLE & UPLIFTING BATH SALTS

What You Will Need:

1 cup Sea Salt

1 tablespoon Baking Soda

3 drops Bergamot essential oil

3 drops Rose Geranium oil

3 drops Lavender essential oil

2 drops Frankincense essential oil

Natural Food Coloring (your choice)

What To Do:

1. In a bowl, add sea salts and baking soda. Add food coloring such as light green or yellow. Stir well.
2. Mix the essential oils in a separate bowl. Pour into the salts and mix well.
3. Store in a clear jar, preferably with a cork-top lid. These are great for gift giving.

EUPHORIC BATH SALTS

Try these oils for an euphoric bath: Clary Sage, Grapefruit, Jasmine absolute, Linden absolute, Myrrh, Patchouli, Rose, and Ylang Ylang.

What You Will Need:

3 tablespoons Sea Salt, or

2 tablespoons Epsom Salt and 1 tablespoon Sea Salt, or

1 tablespoon Powdered Red Earth Clay and 2 tablespoons Sea Salt, or

1 tablespoon Powdered Kelp and 2 tablespoons Sea Salt

3 tablespoons Baking Soda

8 drops essential oils

4-ounce jar

What To Do:

1. Choose a carrier salt.
2. Choose 3-4 oils from the list above.
3. In a jar, add salts, baking soda and essential oils. Gently shake to mix well.
4. To use, add to a tub of running water.

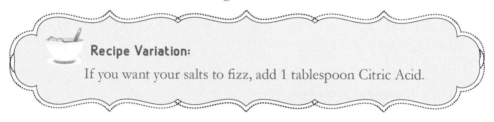

Recipe Variation:

If you want your salts to fizz, add 1 tablespoon Citric Acid.

EARTH ANGEL BATH CRYSTALS

What You Will Need:

½ cup Epsom Salt

¾ cup Baking Soda

½ cup Sea Salt

2 teaspoons Sweet Almond oil

20 drops Patchouli essential oil

15 drops Cypress essential oil

5 drops Rose essential oil

Natural Green Food Coloring

What To Do:

1. In a bowl, mix salts and baking soda.
2. Add 1-2 drops of food coloring and mix well.
3. In a separate bowl, mix essential oils then add to salt mixture.
4. To use, add a few heaping tablespoons to your tub.

GREEN EARTH BATH SALTS

What You Will Need:

½ cup Epsom Salt

1 cup Baking Soda

½ cup Sea Salt

½ teaspoon Vitamin E oil

2 teaspoons Sweet Almond oil

20 drops Patchouli essential oil

15 drops Cypress essential oil

5 drops Vetiver essential oil

Natural Green Food Coloring

Jar or container with lid

What To Do:

1. In a bowl, combine Epsom salts, sea salt, and baking soda together.
2. In a separate bowl, combine almond oil, essential oils, vitamin E oil and a few drops of coloring.
3. Add liquid mixture to the salt mixture and stir thoroughly. Store in a jar or container.
4. To use, add a few heaping tablespoons to a running bath.

DESERT SANDS LAYERED BATH SALTS

What You Will Need:

5 drops Natural Yellow Food Coloring

4 drops Natural Red Food Coloring

4 drops Sandalwood essential oil

3 drops Jasmine essential oil

3 cups Epsom Salt

1 cup Baking Soda

2 teaspoons Glycerin

Jar or container with lid

What To Do:

1. In a bowl, combine baking soda, Epsom salt and glycerin until well blended.

2. Add essential oils and stir until there are no clumps, just a fine powder.

3. Divide the mixture evenly into 3 separate bowls. In the first bowl add 3 drops of yellow food coloring, in the second bowl add 3 drops of red food coloring and in the third bowl add 2 drops of yellow food coloring and 1 drop red food coloring. Stir each bowl until the color is well mixed.

4. Allow the salts to air-dry for a few hours before placing in a bottle. Once dried, layer the colors—red first, then orange, and lastly yellow.

5. Package in a nice jar or container and add a gift tag to give as a gift.

BALANCING BATH SALTS

These oils are great for balancing: Bergamot, Frankincense, Geranium, Lavender, Palmarosa, Rose, and Rosewood. Choose from this list for an incredible bathing experience.

What You Will Need:

3 tablespoons Sea Salt, or

2 tablespoons Epsom Salt and 1 tablespoon Sea Salt, or

1 tablespoon Powdered Red Earth Clay and 2 tablespoons Sea Salt, or

1 tablespoon Powdered Kelp and 2 tablespoons Sea Salt

3 tablespoons Baking Soda

8 drops Essential oils (your choice)

Jar or container with lid

What To Do:

1. Choose a carrier salt.

2. Choose 3-4 oils from the list above.

3. Add salts, baking soda and essential oils to a jar. If you want your salts to fizz, add 1 tablespoon citric acid. Gently shake to mix well.

4. To use, add to a tub of running water.

BASIL & LIME BATH SALTS

What You Will Need:

5 cups of Sea Salt (or Epsom Salt, or a combination of both)

1 teaspoon Baking Powder

2 teaspoon Sweet Almond oil

5 drops Lime essential oil

4 drops Basil essential oil

1 drop Natural Green Food Coloring

1 drop Natural Yellow Food Coloring

Bottle or jar with cork lid

What To Do:

1. In a bowl, mix the salt and the baking powder.
2. In another bowl, add essential oils and food colorings, stirring well. Add to the salt mixture and blend well.
3. Allow mixture to sit for a couple of hours so it can soak up the scent and coloring completely through.
4. Pour the salts into a jar or bottle with a cork stopper. To create a good seal, dip the cork in melted wax and place cork into bottle.

CANDY CANE BATH SALTS

What You Will Need:

3 cups Epsom Salt

3 teaspoons Sweet Almond oil

9 drops Peppermint essential oil

1 drop Natural Red Food Coloring

1 drop Natural Green Food Coloring

Jars with lids

Red, green or white ribbon

Gift tags (shaped like candy canes)

3 bowls

What To Do:

1. Add 1 cup of salt to three separate bowls.

2. Add 1 teaspoon of almond oil to each of the three bowls.

3. In one bowl, add red food coloring. In the second bowl, add green food coloring. Leave the third bowl white.

4. Add three drops of Peppermint oil to each bowl. Stir to mix salts, almond oil, and Peppermint oil. Let sit for a few hours covered.

5. To create the candy cane effect, pour a layer of each colored salt into a jar, alternating the colors, until the jar is filled.

6. Replace lid and tie a colored ribbon around the lid. Add a gift tag to give someone for the holidays.

SINUS HEADACHE BATH SALTS

This is a great relief for a stuffy head.

What You Will Need:

2 cups Epsom Salt (or salts of your choice)

1/3 cup Peppermint leaves

1/3 cup Spearmint leaves

12 drops Peppermint essential oil

12 drops Eucalyptus essential oil

Container with lid

What To Do:

1. Grind the mint leaves with a mortar and pestle then sift them through a kitchen strainer.

2. In a bowl, add salts and mint leaves.

3. Next, stir in the essential oils, one at a time. Blend well.

4. To use, add about ¼-½ cup of this mixture to the bath.

STIMULATING BATH SALTS

For a stimulating bath, use these essential oils: Angelica, Basil, Bay, Black Pepper, Cajeput, Cardamom, Cinnamon, Citronella, Clove, Eucalyptus, Fennel,

Fir, Ginger, Grapefruit, Juniper, Lavender, Lemon, Lemongrass, Nutmeg, Peppermint, Pine, Rosemary, Spearmint, Spruce, Tea Tree, and Thyme.

What You Will Need:

3 tablespoons Sea Salt, or

2 tablespoons Epsom Salt and 1 tablespoon Sea Salt, or

1 tablespoon Powdered Red Earth Clay and 2 tablespoons Sea Salt, or

1 tablespoon Powdered Kelp and 2 tablespoons Sea Salt

3 tablespoons Baking Soda

8 drops Essential oil (your choice)

4-ounce jar

What To Do:

1. Choose a carrier salt.
2. Choose 3-4 oils from the list above.
3. Add salts, baking soda and essential oils to a jar. If you want your salts to fizz, add 1 tablespoon citric acid. Gently shake to mix well.
4. To use, add to a tub of running water.

SUMMER BREEZE BATH SALTS

What You Will Need:

3 cups Epsom Salt

1 cup Baking Soda

9 drops Jasmine essential oil

12 drops Vanilla essential oil

4 drops Sandalwood essential oil

10 drops Natural Blue Food Coloring

Jar with a tight fitting lid

What To Do:

1. In a bowl, add essential oils and food coloring. Blend well.
2. Add the salts and baking soda and blend thoroughly. Let sit for about an hour. Stir one more time before placing the salts in a jar and sealing.
3. To use, add ¼-½ cup to a running bath.

BUTTERMILK BATH SALTS

What You Will Need:

1 cup Buttermilk Powder

1 cup Sea Salt

24 drops Essential oil (your choice)

Bowl

What To Do:

1. In a bowl, add buttermilk powder and sea salt.
2. Add up to 24 drops of essential oils. Blend well. Store in a sealed jar.
3. To use, add ½ cup per bath. This makes enough for 4 baths.

MOONLIGHT SHADOWS BATH SALTS

What You Will Need:

3 cups Epsom Salt

2 cups Baking Soda

1 cup Sea Salt

4 drops Lavender essential oil

4 drops Lily of the Valley essential oil

2 drops Sandalwood essential oil

1 drop Frankincense essential oil

Natural Food Coloring (optional)

Bowl

Jar or container with lid

What To Do:

1. In a bowl, mix together the salts and baking soda.
2. Add the essential oils and coloring into the salt mixture. Blend well.
3. To use, add ½ cup per bath.

VELVET SEDUCTION SALT GLOW

What You Will Need:

¼ cup Kosher Salt

¼ cup Epsom Salt

¼ cup Sea Salt

2 ounces Hazelnut or Jojoba oil

4 drops Rose essential oil

8 drops Sandalwood essential oil

4 drops Ylang Ylang essential oil

Jar or container with lid

What To Do:

1. In a bowl, add Hazelnut or Jojoba oil with the essential oils and mix well.
2. Add the salts to the oils and stir well. Store in jar or container with a lid until ready to use.
3. To use, add ¼-½ cup to a running bath.

ECHOES OF THE WILD BODY BUFFER

What You Will Need:

¼ cup Jojoba oil

¼ cup Liquid soap

½ cup Sea Salt

5 drops Orange essential oil

4 drops Sandalwood essential oil

3 drops Jasmine essential oil

Squeeze Bottle

What To Do:

1. Combine all of the ingredients in a small bowl and mix thoroughly.
2. Pour into a flip-top bottle. This scrub will have a liquid consistency.
3. Use as normal.

CHOCOLATE MILK BATH SALTS

What You Will Need:

1/8 cup Unsweetened Cocoa Powder

1/8 cup Powdered Milk

¼ cup Epsom Salt

1 tablespoon Baking Soda

1 tablespoon Cornstarch

2 drops Peppermint essential oil

What To Do:

1. In a bowl, mix all of the ingredients and stir well.
2. Pour into a warm bath as it is running. This works great in a whirlpool tub too, because it gets frothy and foamy!

CUSTOM-SCENTED BATH SALTS

What You Will Need:

½-1 cup Epsom Salt

½-1 cup Sea Salt

1 tablespoon Baking Soda

5-10 drops Essential oils (your choice)

What To Do:

1. In a bowl, mix all of the ingredients and stir well.
2. Pour into warm bath water as it is running.

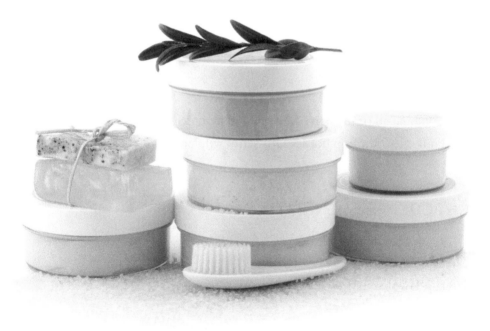

Bath Salt Tips

- Essential oils to avoid in the bath include spicy or warm oils such as Cinnamon, Clove, Black Pepper, Oregano, and Thyme.

  Oils with specific irritant potential and certain phototoxic oils such as citruses should be used with caution.

- Essential oils that are generally considered mild and safe for the bath include: Lavender, Clary Sage, Rose, Geranium, Frankincense, Sandalwood, Eucalyptus, and conifers such as Cedarwood, Balsam Fir, Pine, Spruce, and Juniper, to name a few.

- A generally safe dose of essential oils in the bath is 5-10 drops, mixed with ½-1 cup of salt or emulsifier.

- Keep in mind: try not to overuse essential oils in the bath, as they may cause irritation.

- Stick to only mild, non-irritating oils for bath, such as Lavender and Clary Sage.

Bubble Baths

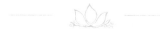

These bubble bath recipes are not only easy to make but beat the over-priced store-bought ones by a mile! And if you do not have a bathtub, don't worry! You can use these homemade bubble baths as a body cleanser as well, so feel free to use these in the shower.

All of the recipes included here call for an essential oil. Just add a few drops to your bubble bath recipe and you're good to go! Feel free to substitute another essential oil and experiment with different fragrances. As you probably know, different oils offer varying purposes.

Try not to skip on adding the glycerin to your bubble bath concoction. This is what makes your skin feel soft and smooth because it attracts water molecules keeping your skin moisturized. It is also what aids in the formation of bubbles. Every bubble bath needs lots of bubbles, of course!

FLOWER CHILD BUBBLE BATH

What You Will Need:

16 ounces Organic Unscented Shampoo

1 bunch Fresh Lavender flowers

5 drops Lavender essential oil

Quart-sized canning jar

Strainer

Bottle

Jar with lid

What To Do:

1. Tie the Lavender flowers in a bunch and place head first in the canning jar, so that the stems are at the top.
2. Now pour the unscented shampoo over the lavender flowers in the jar.
3. Add 5 drops of Lavender essential oil.
4. Close the lid securely and give the jar a good shake. Leave the mixture to rest on a sunny window sill for about two weeks. Shake the jar everyday while it is sitting.
5. At the end of the two-week period, strain the mixture and pour your bubble bath liquid into a bottle.

SURF'S UP BUBBLE BATH

What You Will Need:

8 ounces Organic Unscented Liquid Soap

2 ounces Distilled Water

7 drops Bergamot essential oil

5 drops Lime essential oil

3 drops Vanilla essential oil

2 drops Gardenia essential oil

Jar or container with lid

What To Do:

1. Mix the liquid soap, water and essential oils together.
2. Pour mixture into a covered container until ready for use.

TROPICAL PARADISE BUBBLE SOAK

Visions of beaches and tropical sunsets will dance through your head as you soak in this luxurious bath.

What You Will Need:

3 drops Rose essential oil

2 drops Jasmine essential oil

4 drops Bergamot essential oil

3 drops Lime essential oil

1 ounce Glycerin

1 ounce Coconut oil

1 bar Castile soap (grated)

1 quart Distilled Water

Container with lid

What To Do:

1. Mix all of the ingredients together and store in a container.
2. To use, pour ½ cup of the bubble bath solution into the flow of running bath water.

ENCHANTED FOREST BUBBLE BATH

What You Will Need:

1 quart Distilled Water

1 bar Castile soap, grated

3 ounces Glycerin

2 drops Pine essential oil

4 drops Spruce essential oil

5 drops Cypress essential oil

2 drops Cedarwood essential oil

Bottle

What To Do:

1. Mix all of the ingredients together and store in a container.
2. To use, pour ½ cup of the bubble bath solution into the flow of running bath water.

ROSY RED BUBBLING BATH

What You Will Need:

1 bar Castile soap, grated

3 ounces Glycerin

1 quart Distilled Water

5 drops Rose essential oil

What To Do:

1. Thoroughly blend all of the ingredients together.
2. Store in a decorative bottle or jar.
3. Shake well before each use and pour about ¼ cup under the flow of your warm running bath water.

SWEET DREAMS BUBBLE BATH

With Lavender and Patchouli's relaxing effects, this bubble bath is great to use before bed. Add soft music and small tea light candles in your bathroom for a soothing effect.

What You Will Need:

6 drops Lavender essential oil

3 drops Patchouli essential oil

1 quart Distilled Water

4-ounce bar Castile soap

4 ounces Glycerin

What To Do:

1. Mix the water, soap and glycerin together and stir well.
2. Add your essential oils to the mixture.
3. Store in bottle or container until ready to use.

COLD SEASON BUBBLE BATH

Use this bubble bath during cold and flu season. With Eucalyptus, Spearmint, and Peppermint essential oils, this one works great for loosening congestion and breathing easier.

What You Will Need:

6 drops Eucalyptus essential oil

3 drops Spearmint essential oil

3 drops Peppermint essential oil

1 quart Distilled Water

4-ounce bar Castile soap

4 ounces Glycerin

Jar or container

What To Do:

1. Mix the water, soap and liquid glycerin together and stir.
2. Add your essential oils to the mixture. Store in a jar or sealed container until ready for use.
3. To use, pour into a warm running bath.

DON'T WORRY, BE HAPPY BATH

This citrusy bubble bath is great for after a workout or on a gloomy, rainy day. The essential oils of Orange, Grapefruit, and Lemon will cheer you up and give you energy.

What You Will Need:

6 drops Orange essential oil

4 drops Grapefruit essential oil

3 drops Lemon essential oil

1 quart Distilled Water

4-ounce bar Castile soap

4 ounces Glycerin

What To Do:

1. Mix the water, soap and glycerin together and stir.
2. Add your essential oils to the mixture. Store in a closed jar or container.
3. To use, pour into a bath of running water.

LOVE POTION BUBBLE BATH

This bubble bath will put you in a romantic mood. All of the ingredients are considered known aphrodisiacs—so look out!

What You Will Need:

6 drops Jasmine essential oil

3 drops Rose essential oil

3 drops Vanilla essential oil

6 drops Ylang Ylang essential oil

1 quart Distilled Water

4 ounces Castile soap

4 ounces Glycerin

What To Do:

1. Mix the water, soap and glycerin together and stir.
2. Add your essential oils to the mixture.

CUSTOM-SCENTED BUBBLE BATH

What You Will Need:

5 drops Essential oil (your choice)

1 quart Distilled Water

1 bar Castile soap (grated or flaked)

1 ½ ounces Glycerin

What To Do:

1. Mix all ingredients together in a large container.
2. When ready to use, pour in a running warm bath.

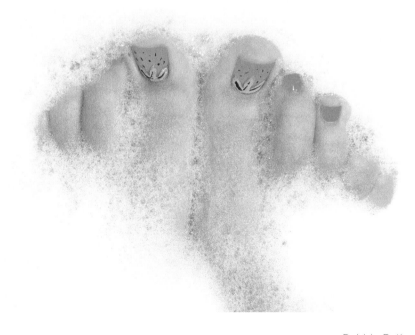

Bubble Bath Tips

- Peppermint, Spearmint, Eucalyptus and Lemon are all essential oils that will brighten your day and are good for daytime use.
- Eucalyptus essential oil is especially good in the bath when you have a cold because it breaks up your cold's congestion.
- For a soothing and relaxing bath use essential oils such as Lavender, Roman and German Chamomile, Sandalwood, Jasmine or Rosewood. These oils can help you get a better night's sleep.
- For a more invigorating bath, try adding Rosemary, Tea Tree, Bergamot, Ginger, Clary Sage, or Basil essential oil.
- To lift your spirits and gain energy, try using Lemon, Spearmint, Peppermint, or Eucalyptus essential oil.
- To soften your skin, consider adding either Coconut or Sweet Almond oil to your bubble bath concoctions. Coconut oil has a wonderful nutty and floral fragrance to it. Sweet Almond oil is virtually unscented. Adding a half a cup oft either Sweet Almond oil or Coconut oil to your bubble bath will soften your skin tremendously. This is a great addition to your bubble baths for the winter months.
- Store your bubble bath in a non-breakable container on a shelf in your bathroom for easy access.

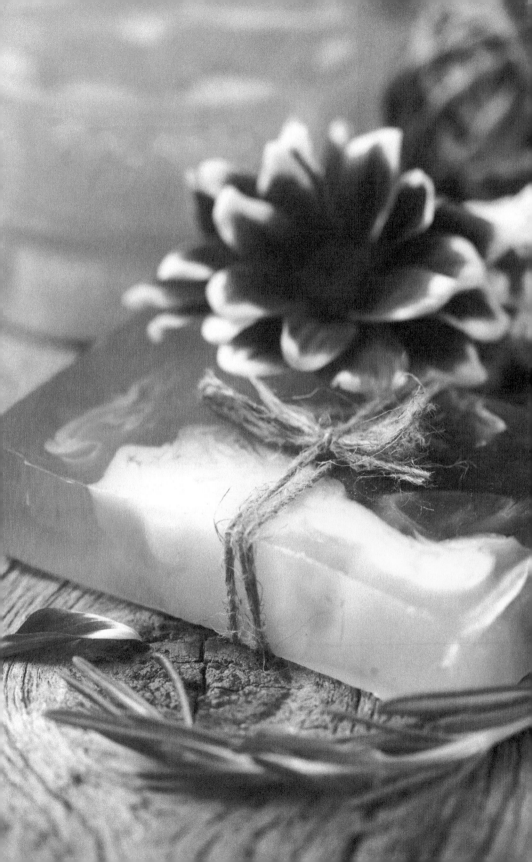

Bath Soaps

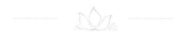

Discover skin indulgences in your bath! Bath soaps drenched with essential oils and moisturizing lotion bars filled with beautiful aromas are good for your skin, leaving it smooth and soft.

Using melt and pour soap bases may seem like cheating a bit when it comes to making homemade soap, but it is one of the safest ways to start for beginners. It is so easy, even the kids can do it!

You can melt the soap base either in a double boiler or microwave. If you use the double boiler method, simply add the melt and pour in and heat on low until the soap contents have melted. When using the microwave, cover your dish with plastic wrap to keep from losing moisture, and heat on high in 30-second increments until soap is completely melted. Stir well to get remaining pieces mixed in.

Next, add your essential oils to the soap base and blend. A general rule of thumb for fragrant essential oils is ¼ ounce per pound but you can adjust as needed, depending on the essential oil you use. To add color, just stir in ¼ teaspoon of mica or a drop or two of natural food coloring into the melted base. Careful though; you don't want to end up with stained hands or hand towels after using your soap. Spray your soap molds with non-stick cooking spray to prevent sticking. While the soap base is still hot, pour into a mold, and spray any bubbles that may have surfaced with alcohol. Once the soap has hardened, remove the bar from its mold. In just a few hours, your soaps are ready!

BUSY BEE SOAP

What You Will Need:

4 ounces Opaque Melt and Pour soap base

1 tablespoon Beeswax

1 tablespoon Honey

10 drops Orange essential oil

Plastic mold

Cooking spray

What To Do:

1. Spray mold with cooking spray to prevent sticking.
2. Melt the beeswax and keep warm, in a liquid state.
3. Melt the soap base and pour into the beeswax.
4. Add honey and keep stirring until melted.
5. Add your essential oils. Pour into mold and allow to sit until they have hardened.

LEMON LOOFAH SOAP

What You Will Need:

Dried Loofah sponge

4 ounces Transparent Melt and Pour soap base

1 teaspoon Liquid Lanolin

1 teaspoon Aloe Vera gel

15 drops Lemon essential oil

1 drop Natural Yellow Food Coloring

Cooking spray

Mold

What To Do:

1. Spray mold with cooking spray to prevent sticking.
2. With a pair of sharp scissors, cut off 1 square inch of the Loofah sponge. Shred the Loofah sponge into tiny pieces, either in a coffee grinder or with scissors, and set aside.

3. Melt the Melt and Pour soap base. Remove from heat.

4. Add the lanolin, Aloe Vera gel, Lemon essential oil, and natural food coloring, stirring until well mixed.

5. Immediately add the shredded Loofah and stir until evenly distributed. Pour into a mold and let set for 3 hours or until hardened. Makes one 4-ounce bar.

LAVENDER CITRUS SOAP

What You Will Need:

2 cups Grated soap

½ cup Water

6 capsules Vitamin E oil (or 15-18 drops)

1 tablespoon Dried Lemon Verbena leaves, ground

1 tablespoon Dried Lavender buds

10 drops Lavender essential oil

20 drops Orange essential oil

What To Do:

1. In a pan, melt the soap with water. After it has melted, add the remaining ingredients.

2. When the soap has cooled and thickened, scoop out a small handful of the soap and roll into a ball. Flatten the ball to create a disk shape. As the soap cures, press the soap into a firmer and smoother shape.

3. Sprinkle a few drops of Orange essential oil onto your hands and polish the soap smooth.

Note: This soap will discolor if the Lavender buds are added too soon to the melted soap. If you do not like the rough surface and the darkened color, omit the Lavender buds. After a week of curing, you can slice thin shavings from the soap to smooth it and remove any dark patches.

CAMPHOR & CLARY SAGE SOAP

Great for poison ivy and other skin irritations!

What You Will Need:

2 cups Opaque Melt and Pour soap base

2 tablespoons Camphor essential oil

1 teaspoon Clary Sage essential oil

Mold

Cooking spray

What To Do:

1. Spray mold with cooking spray to prevent sticking.
2. In a pan, heat the Melt and Pour base. Add essential oils and stir until blended.
3. Pour into molds. Keep soap wrapped or store in a cool dark place. It will keep for about 18 months.

SAINT PATTY'S SOAP

Try this refreshing soap for sore muscles.

What You Will Need:

2 cups Opaque Melt and Pour soap base

1 bag Celestial Seasonings Spearmint tea

5-6 drops Natural Green Food Coloring

1 teaspoon Wintergreen essential oil

What To Do:

1. Heat the Melt and Pour soap in a double boiler or microwave until melted.
2. While it is heating, open the tea bag and grind the leaves in a coffee grinder or pestle.
3. Add the ground leaves, Wintergreen essential oil and natural food coloring to the melted soap and stir.
4. Pour into shamrock shaped molds and let cool. Voila—St. Paddy's Day soap!

WEEKEND IN TIJUANA SOAP

What You Will Need:

8 ounces Transparent Melt and Pour soap base

2 tablespoons Cornmeal

1 ½ tablespoon Fine Pumice

1 tablespoon Bentonite Clay

6-8 drops Cilantro essential oil

6-8 drops Lime essential oil

Mold

Cooking spray

What To Do:

1. Spray mold with cooking spray to prevent sticking.
2. In a glass measuring cup, melt the Melt and Pour soap base in a double boiler or microwave for 30-second increments until melted.
3. Add in essential oils. Stir in cornmeal, pumice, and clay until it reaches the point where it will stay suspended in the soap. By this time the soap will be quite thick and cool.
4. Pour into molds and allow to sit until hardened.

BUG OFF CITRONELLA SOAP

What You Will Need:

1 cup Grated Castile soap

½ cup Water

10 drops Citronella essential oil

5 drops Eucalyptus essential oil

1 tablespoon dried Pennyroyal leaves, crushed

Mold

Cooking spray

What To Do:

1. Spray mold with cooking spray to prevent sticking.
2. In a pan, melt the soap with the water.

3. Add all of the ingredients into the melted soap/water mixture.
4. With an electric mixer, whip the soap until it has doubled in volume.
5. Spoon the soap into the prepared molds, pushing it into the molds as best you can (the beating action cools the mix, so work quickly). If the mixture has cooled off and thickened so much you can't put it into the molds, hand mold the soap into large balls.

FAT ATTACK SOAP

Just like the name suggests, the essential oils in this soap help to eliminate fat and cellulite in the body. Scrub, ladies, scrub!

What You Will Need:

½ pound Transparent Melt and Pour soap base

½ tablespoon Coconut oil

3 drops Lemon essential oil

3 drops Grapefruit essential oil

3 drops Orange essential oil

Fruit wedge molds

1-2 drops Natural Orange Food Coloring

1-2 drops Natural Yellow Food Coloring

Cooking spray

What To Do:

1. Spray mold with cooking spray to prevent sticking.
2. Melt the soap base and coconut oil in a pan. Remove from heat and whisk well.
3. Add the essential oils and stir well. Add in a few drops of natural food coloring.
4. Pour into molds.

MINT & EUCALYPTUS COLD CREAM SOAP

What You Will Need:

4 ounces Opaque Melt and Pour soap base

2 teaspoons Cold Cream

5 drops Eucalyptus essential oil

5 drops Peppermint essential oil

1 drop Natural Green Food Coloring (optional)

Mold

Cooking spray

What To Do:

1. Spray mold with cooking spray to prevent sticking.
2. Melt the soap base in a pan, then add cold cream and stir until melted.
3. Remove from heat; add essential oils and natural food coloring of choice.
4. Pour into a mold and let sit for several hours. It is best if allowed to cure for 3-7 days.

CREAMY ROSEMARY SOAP

This is a wonderfully creamy soap to wake up to in the morning! Everyone loves the scent of pure Rosemary—even men!

What You Will Need:

1 pound Melt and Pour soap base

1 cup Whole Milk

½ teaspoon Rosemary essential oil

1 foot-long PVC pipe with end cap

What To Do:

1. Spray the inside of your PVC pipe mold with a vegetable cooking spray.
2. Heat the soap base and add the milk and essential oil.
3. Pour the soap mixture into the pipe. After a couple of hours, push it out and slice the soap into round soaps!
4. Warning: Rosemary essential oil is not recommended for individuals with high blood pressure or epilepsy.

HOT MAMA CINNAMON SOAP

What You Will Need:

4 ounces Melt and Pour soap base

10 drops Cinnamon essential oil

1 drop Natural Red Food Coloring (optional)

Mold

Cooking spray

What To Do:

1. Spray mold with cooking spray to prevent sticking.
2. Dissolve Melt and Pour soap base in a pan on the stovetop or microwave.
3. Remove from heat and stir in the Cinnamon oil and natural food coloring until well mixed.
4. Pour the soap into a mold and let set for 3 hours. Let bars cure for several days.

CITRUS & CALENDULA SOAP

This very pretty soap is great for gifts.

What You Will Need:

1 pound Transparent Melt and Pour soap base

¼ cup Dried Calendula petals (dried)

15 drops Natural Yellow Food Coloring

¾ teaspoon Grapefruit essential oil

½ teaspoon Tangerine essential oil

1 tablespoon Shea butter, melted

Heart-shape molds

Cooking spray

What To Do:

1. Spray molds with cooking spray to prevent sticking.
2. Melt the soap base and Shea butter in separate custard cups placed in a pan of boiling water or in the microwave.
3. Add calendula petals, a few drops of yellow food coloring, and essential oils into the melted soap base.
4. Add the melted Shea butter. Keep stirring the soap/Shea butter mixture to prevent the butter from floating to the top and making little circles on the surface.

5. As it starts to set, spoon into heart molds. (By spooning you have more control how many calendula leaves go into each mold.)
6. Let the soaps set at room temperature until they are fairly firm, then chill in the freezer for about a half hour before removing them from the mold.
7. Place soaps on a rack to finish drying completely. Makes 8 heart soaps.

LOTION BARS (SOLID BATH OIL BARS)

These bars have multiple uses. After showering you can rub on the body like the elbows and knees while still damp, or massage into cuticles to soften them. You can even place one in a drawer as a sachet, or cut off a sliver and let melt in hot bath water. Add a bit more carrier oil to this recipe for a softer bar—great for massages.

What You Will Need:

2 ounces Deodorized Cocoa or Mango butter

2 ounces Beeswax

2-3 ounces Carrier oil (such as Jojoba, Sunflower, or Sweet Almond)

2 teaspoons Essential oil (your choice)

Glass measuring cup

What To Do:
1. In a microwave, melt cocoa or mango butter and beeswax and pour into an 8-ounce glass measuring cup.
2. Add 2 ounces carrier oil to mixture. If you prefer a softer bar, add 3 ounces.
3. Stir thoroughly. Add essential oils once mixture has cooled slightly.
4. Pour into small soap molds. Pop out when cool, about 2 hours. For best results, put in refrigerator a few minutes before popping out of mold.

CREAMSICLE SOAP

What You Will Need:

8 ounces Melt and Pour soap base

10 drops Orange essential oil

1 drop Natural Orange Food Coloring

3 tablespoons Heavy Whipping Cream

10 drops Vanilla essential oil

Molds

Cooking spray

What To Do:

1. Spray cooking spray on molds to prevent sticking.
2. Melt 4 ounces of the soap and remove from heat.
3. Add the Orange essential oil and natural food coloring, stirring until well mixed.
4. Pour mixture into each soap mold, filling halfway, and let it set for 1 hour.
5. When the orange soap has set, melt the other 4 ounces of soap and remove from heat.
6. Stir in the whipping cream and the Vanilla essential oil.
7. Pour mixture into the molds on top of the orange soap. Let it set for 3 hours. Your finished bars should come out half orange and half white. Makes 2 bars.

CHAMOMILE & OATS SOAP

What You Will Need:

1/3 cup Dried Oats

4 ounces Melt and Pour soap base

15 drops German Chamomile essential oil

1 drop Natural Red Food Coloring (optional)

Mold

Cooking spray

What To Do:

1. Spray mold with cooking spray to prevent sticking.
2. Grind the oats into a fine powder in a food processor and set aside.
3. Melt the Melt and Pour soap base. Remove from heat and add the Orange essential oil, the natural food coloring, and oat powder, stirring until well mixed.
4. Pour into a soap mold and let set for 3 hours or until hardened.

DOUBLE MINT SOAP

What You Will Need:

1 pound Melt and Pour soap base

1 tablespoon Mint leaves (finely crushed)

½ teaspoon Peppermint essential oil

½ teaspoon Spearmint essential oil

Mold

Cooking spray

What To Do:

1. Spray mold with cooking spray to prevent sticking.
2. Melt soap base in a microwave in a glass measuring cup.
3. Add mint leaves and essential oils.
4. Pour into molds and let set for 3 hours or until hardened.

MAMA ROSA'S COLD CREAM SOAP

This old-fashion recipe will bring back memories of Grandma's rose garden!

What You Will Need:

4 ounces Opaque Melt and Pour soap base

2 teaspoons Cold Cream

10 drops Rose essential oil

1 drop Natural Red Food Coloring (optional)

Mold

Cooking spray

What To Do:

1. In a pan, melt the Melt and Pour soap base until liquefied.
2. Stir in the cold cream until dissolved and remove the pan from heat.
3. Stir in the Rose essential oil and natural food coloring. Blend well.
4. Pour into mold and let set for 4 hours or until hardened. Makes 1 bar.

WILD GARDEN SHOWER SOAP

What You Will Need:

½ cup Distilled Water

½ cup Orange Floral water

1 tablespoons Peppermint leaves, dried, or

5 drops Peppermint essential oil

1 tablespoon Roman Chamomile, dried or

5 drops Roman Chamomile essential oil

1 tablespoon Rose petals, dried

1 tablespoon Orange blossoms, or

1 teaspoon Orange essential oil

½-1 tablespoon Glycerin soap, unscented

What To Do:

1. Combine the distilled water and Orange floral water in a saucepan and bring to a boil.

2. Remove the pan from heat and add the Peppermint, Chamomile, Rose petals, and Orange blossoms. Let steep for 1 hour.

3. Strain the herbs and flowers from the water and reheat gently. Add the glycerin soap and stir. Let the mixture cool to room temperature and pour into a bottle.

SEA SALT & PEPPER SOAP

What You Will Need:

½ pound White Glycerin soap

½ pound Clear Glycerin soap

½ tablespoon Salt

½ tablespoon Castor oil

½ tablespoon Beeswax

¼ cup Sea Salt

2 tablespoons Poppy Seeds

¼ teaspoon Black Pepper essential oil

1 teaspoon Peppercorns, crushed

What To Do:

1. Melt the clear soap in a double boiler or in the microwave in a glass measuring cup.
2. Add table salt to melted soap base.
3. Pour into a rectangle-shaped mold so soap will be approximately ¼ inch thick.
4. Sprinkle sea salt on top. When it cools, cut into triangular shapes and place pieces into another mold.
5. Melt white glycerin in a double boiler or in a microwave in a glass measuring cup.
6. Add castor oil, beeswax, poppy seeds, peppercorns and essential oil to melted soap base.
7. Pour over clear, sea salt soap triangles.
8. Let cool, then remove from molds.

SILKY SMOOTH BATH WASH

What You Will Need:

8 drops Jasmine essential oil

8 drops Fennel essential oil

2 tablespoons Coconut or Jojoba oil

What To Do:

1. Pour carrier oil and essential oils into the palm of your hand and stir with finger to blend.
2. Add oils to a running, warm bath. Swish around in tub to mix well. Light a candle and relax.

SOAP OF THE MAGI

These soaps are scented with the heavenly combination of Frankincense and Myrrh. The spicy, woody scent of Frankincense is uplifting, while the balsamic, musky scent of Myrrh is known to be anti-fungal and healing. These beautiful gems serve as reminders of the gifts that the Magi brought to the Messiah.

What You Will Need:

5 ounces Opaque Melt and Pour soap base

1/8 teaspoon Myrrh essential oil

1/8 teaspoon Frankincense essential oil

Bronze and Gold mica dust

Ultra fine gold fabric glitter

Oval soap mold

What To Do:

1. Melt half of the soap.
2. Stir in the Frankincense essential oil and gold mica dust. Pour into molds, filling half way.
3. Melt the other half of the soap.
4. Stir in the Myrrh essential oil and bronze mica dust.
5. Spoon over first layer of soap. Let set, and unmold.
6. Give the bars a light dusting of the gold glitter.
7. Give as gifts for the holidays.

THYME FOR LEMON SOAP

This is a sweet-scented soap with strong anti-bacterial properties.

What You Will Need:

2 pounds Transparent Melt and Pour soap base

2 teaspoons Coconut oil

1 tablespoon Lemon essential oil

1 teaspoon Thyme essential oil

4 teaspoons Thyme leaves, dried

2 teaspoons Lemon peels, grated

Yellow Natural Food Coloring

Molds

What To Do:

1. In a pan, melt your soap base. Stir in the coconut oil. Set aside and let cool for a few minutes.

2. Add in the essential oils, lemon peels and thyme leaves.

3. Pour into your mold. As your soap starts to thicken, stir once more to make sure the lemon peels and thyme leaves are evenly distributed throughout the soap.

4. Let harden, unmold, cut and use.

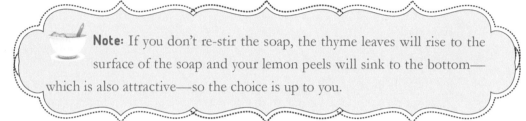

Note: If you don't re-stir the soap, the thyme leaves will rise to the surface of the soap and your lemon peels will sink to the bottom—which is also attractive—so the choice is up to you.

BASIL & BERGAMOT SOAP

This recipe gives you an eco-friendly soap with a penetrating herbal aroma of Basil and Bergamot.

What You Will Need:

1 pounds and 1 ounces Transparent Melt and Pour soap

½ tablespoon Apricot Kernel oil

½ teaspoon Basil essential oil

½ teaspoon Bergamot essential oil

1 teaspoons Lavender essential oil

½ tablespoon Calendula petals

2 teaspoons Basil leaves

1-2 drops Orange or Yellow Natural Food Coloring

Molds

What To Do:

1. In a microwave or stovetop, melt your soap base, stirring in your Apricot oil. Remove from heat and let cool for a few minutes.

2. Stir in the essential oils.

3. Add a small amount of natural food coloring to make it orange or until desired shade is achieved.

4. Coarsely grind your Basil and Calendula petals and stir them into your soap base.
5. Pour into your molds and let harden. Once hard, unmold and cut into bars.

MASSAGE MELTS

Honey works very well in these massage bars, leaving no sticky feeling. However, if you prefer a softer bar use a carrier oil such as Sweet Almond or Jojoba instead.

What You Will Need:

2 tablespoons Beeswax

2 tablespoons Cocoa butter

1 tablespoon Honey, or

1½ teaspoons Carrier oil (Palm, Olive, Almond, or Jojoba)

5-10 drops Essential oil (your choice)

What To Do:

1. Melt the beeswax in a double boiler with water then add the honey (or oil) and whisk together.
2. Add the essential oil and blend well.
3. Be sure to keep the beeswax very hot while mixing. Pour into mold and let set overnight in the refrigerator.

MECHANIC'S HAND CLEANSER

Don't forget to put a nail brush and pumice stone out with the hand cleanser.

What You Will Need:

1 cup Borax Powder

1-2 teaspoons Pine essential oil

1 teaspoon Orange essential oil

1 cup Soap, ground

What To Do:

1. With very clean hands, work the Pine and Orange essential oils into the Borax until there are no lumps.

2. Next, work in the soap. Store in a wide-mouthed jar or tin that's easy to open.

CUSTOM-SCENTED GLYCERIN SOAP

What You Will Need:

1 pound Glycerin soap

1 teaspoon Essential oil (your choice)

1 cup Boiling Water

½ cup Herbs, Rose Petals, Oatmeal, Cornmeal (optional)

¼-½ cup Herbal tea (infusion)

What To Do:

1. Melt the glycerin in a double boiler with water (or herbal infusion).
2. If using powders, stir in with a non-metallic spoon. Let mixture cool slightly (not enough to harden—still pourable) and add the essential oils.
3. Pour into molds or a plastic wrap-lined box.
4. Once hardened, cut into bars and bevel the edges and rough spots with a paring knife. This recipe can also be made with Castile soap flakes.

CUSTOM-SCENTED LIQUID / GEL SOAP

What You Will Need:

2 cups Soap flakes or grated bar soap

½ gallon Water

2 tablespoons Glycerin

1 teaspoon Essential oil (your choice)

Natural Food Coloring (your choice)

What To Do:

1. In a large pot, mix the soap, glycerin, and water together. Set over low heat, stirring occasionally, until the soap has dissolved.
2. Add essential oil and natural food coloring, stirring well. Transfer to a jar and cover tightly. For thinner gel soap, add one gallon of water.

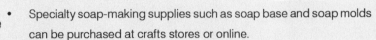

Bath Soap Tips

- Specialty soap-making supplies such as soap base and soap molds can be purchased at crafts stores or online.
- Add a drop or two of natural food coloring to give color to your homemade soap.
- Popular essential oil choices for homemade soap include: Tea Tree (it has anti-bacterial properties and helps clear the skin), Lavender (the smell is relaxing and calming), and citrus oils such as Orange and Lemon (they have invigorating scents).
- To help the soap harden more quickly, place your soap mold in the freezer for 10-15 minutes.
- Be careful when working with hot soap base, as it may cause burns if accidentally spilled on the skin. Dab Lavender essential oil directly on the burn if this happens.

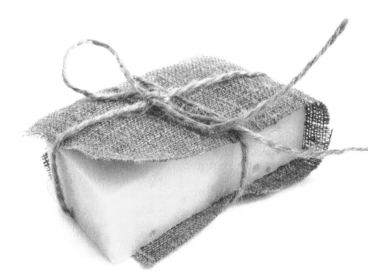

Milk Baths

Aromatic milk baths have been practiced for thousands of years. Cleopatra, Queen of the Nile, was known to indulge herself in fragrant camel and goat milk baths with rose petals everyday to maintain her lavish soft skin. Other royal figures have acclaimed their beauty to this practice as well because of its simple luxury's health benefits. Scientific research has confirmed Cleopatra's wisdom and proven the astounding rejuvenating properties of milk baths with rose petals and Rosehips.

Vitamins A and D found in milk help make your skin soft, while the lactic acid with alpha hydroxyl acids dissolve the sticky proteins that keep dead cells attached to the skin. The lactic acid also acts as a gentle moisturizing exfoliant. By removing this top layer of dead skin, your complexion is improved and blotchy, dull-looking skin is prevented.

The recipes contained in this section are super easy. You can also create your own fragrant milk bath by choosing essential oils that will enhance your mood or other health benefits. You may want to add essential oils that will invigorate, giving you energy, or essential oils for relaxation after a long, hard day at the office. Check the list of essential oils in the chapters entitled, *Essential Oils for Setting the Mood* and *Essential Oils for the Skin* for suggestions.

To create your milk bath, simply add 8-10 drops of therapeutic essential oils such as Lavender, Jasmine, or Rosemary to 1-2 cups of whole or low-fat milk (using dry milk works too). Add to a warm, running bath to distribute the milk mixture. Soak for 15-20 minutes while going over your skin with a Loofah or washcloth in a circular motion. When you are finished, rinse the milk residue off your body in the shower. Afterwards, you will be left with a noticeably silky feel to your skin.

ROSE & HONEY MILK BATH

Both honey and Rose have a long list of health benefits, so together they make a wonderful combination! Soaking in warm milk with just a dab of honey feels ultra-relaxing.

What You Will Need:

1 ½ cups Whole Milk

1/3 cup Honey

5 drops Rose essential oil

What To Do:

1. In a bowl, stir in milk, honey and essential oil.
2. Pour ½ cup of mixture into a warm bath.

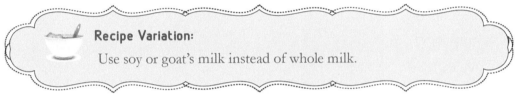

Recipe Variation:

Use soy or goat's milk instead of whole milk.

FIELDS OF GOLD MILK BATH

With Chamomile's anti-bacterial, antiseptic, antibiotic, and vermifuge properties, this bath recipe can really come in handy for when you are not up to speed! This bath is good after a long day in the sun or if you are suffering from poison ivy or poison oak.

What You Will Need:

4 cups Powdered Milk

1 cup Boiled Water

½ cup Dried Chamomile, or 6 Chamomile tea bags

5 drops Roman Chamomile essential oil

1 tablespoon Honey

1 tablespoon Oatmeal

Pan or kettle

What To Do:

1. Steep the dried Chamomile in the water for about 20 minutes. Strain liquid.

2. Add all of the other ingredients to the tea liquid.

3. Pour ½ cup of mixture into the flow of your running bath water.

OATMEAL MILK BATH

Using oatmeal in the bath is one of the oldest remedies for itching or irritated skin. This milk bath is great for those days when you experience over-exposure to the sun or come into contact with poison ivy.

What You Will Need:

½ cup Powdered Milk

¼ cup Oatmeal

1 tablespoon Hazelnut oil

6 drops Lavender essential oil

1 Muslin bag

Small bowl

What To Do:

1. Combine the milk powder, Hazelnut oil and Lavender essential oil in a small bowl and mix thoroughly.

2. Place your oatmeal in a muslin bag and secure the top.

3. While running your bath, add the combined mixture directly under the warm running water then drop the muslin bag of oats straight into the tub and enjoy.

SOOTHING LAVENDER-CHAMOMILE MILK BATH

Known for its soothing and relaxing properties, Lavender is one of the best essential oils to have on hand. Here is a simple recipe for a milk bath gentle enough for children.

What You Will Need:

1 cup Powdered Milk

10 drops Lavender essential oil

9 drops Lemon essential oil

1 drop Roman Chamomile essential oil

Bowl

What To Do:

1. In a bowl, thoroughly mix the essential oils and milk powder.
2. Add to your running bath water and enjoy.

ORIENTAL NIGHTS MILK BATH

The exotic fragrances of Jasmine, Ylang Ylang and Mandarin take you far away!

What You Will Need:

1 cup Powdered Milk

1 tablespoon Orrisroot powder

¾ cup Himalayan salt (fine)

10 drops Jasmine essential oil

7 drops Ylang Ylang essential oil

5 drops Mandarin essential oil

Bowls

Jar with lid

What To Do:

1. In a small bowl, mix the powdered milk, Orrisroot powder and salt.
2. Scoop out ½ cup of powder mixture into another bowl. Add your essential oils and mix well.
3. Add the scented powder mixture to the first bowl of powder mixture and blend well. Store in a glass jar with a tight fitting lid.
4. To use, add ½-1 cup to warm running bath water. Swish around in the bath water to distribute well.

SLEEP EASY TONIGHT BATH

Nothing is better than a warm, relaxing bath before bed!

What You Will Need:

1 teaspoon Milk or Cream

3 drops Lavender essential oil

1 drop Clary Sage essential oil

Spoon

What To Do:

1. Mix all of the ingredients in a bowl.
2. Pour mixture into a warm bath and soak before bed.

EXEC'S STRESS RELIEF MILK BATH

This bath will calm the nerves and promote restful sleep.

What You Will Need:

1 teaspoon Milk or Cream

4 drops Lavender essential oil

4 drops Roman Chamomile essential oil

Spoon

What To Do:

1. Mix all of the ingredients in a bowl.
2. Pour mixture into a warm bath and soak.

NEW MOON MILK BATH

The beginning of each new month is a time of reflection and inwardness. Celebrate in a soothing bath!

What You Will Need:

2 cups Powdered Milk

½ cup Epsom Salt

½ cup Baking Soda

6 drops Sandalwood essential oil

5 drops Vanilla essential oil

4 drops Gardenia absolute oil

4 drops Orange essential oil

Bowl

Jar with lid

What To Do:

1. In a bowl, add all of the dry ingredients and mix well.
2. Stir in each essential oil and blend. Store in a jar with a lid to keep airtight.

3. To use, pour 1 cup of mixture into a running bath and swish to mix thoroughly.

TROPICAL PARADISE MILK BATH

For the perfect tropical bath escape, try this recipe using Coconut milk with Vanilla essential oil!

What You Will Need:

2 cups Coconut Milk

3 drops Lime essential oil

3 drops Ylang Ylang essential oil

6 drops Vanilla essential oil

Fresh flower petals

Bowl

Jar with lid

What To Do:

1. In a bowl, combine the milk and essential oils.
2. Add 1 cup of mixture to a warm running bath.
3. Drop flower petals into water and soak your worries away.

CINNAMON STICK MILK BATH

Indulge yourself in a luxurious chocolate milk bath with Cinnamon and Anise Star essentials oils!

What You Will Need:

1 cup Powdered Milk

1/8 cup Cocoa Powder

1 tablespoon Cornstarch

5 drops Cinnamon essential oil

5 drops Anise Star essential oil

Small bowl

What To Do:

1. Mix all of the ingredients together in a small bowl.

2. As tub is filling, pour ½-1 cup of chocolate mixture in the running bath.
3. Swish around to dissolve in bath. Enjoy!

MINT-CHOCOLATE MILK BATH

Melt into a hot bath with the sweet aroma of Mint and cocoa. This milk bath lavishes your skin leaving a silky softening finish. Light some candles to enhance your quiet time in the tub!

What You Will Need:

2 cups Powdered Milk, or Fresh Milk

5 tablespoons Fresh or Dried Mint leaves

5-10 drops Peppermint essential oil

3 tablespoons Cocoa Powder

½ cup Epsom Salt

1 cup Cornstarch

Bowl

Small jar with lid

What To Do:

1. In a bowl, add all of your dry ingredients. Mix thoroughly.
2. Stir in fresh milk, if using. Add essential oils one drop at a time and stir to blend well.
3. Store the dry mix in a jar for later use or use the liquid mixture immediately in a hot bath.

ROSE & LIME MILK BATH

This unique combination of Rose and Lime is great for oily skin types. Lime works great as an astringent, absorbing excess oil on the skin, reducing acne breakouts, and shrinking pores.

What You Will Need:

3 cups Fresh Milk, or 2 cups Powdered Milk

2 cups Rose Petals

5 drops Rose essential oil

3 Limes

3 drops Lime essential oil

Bowl

What To Do:

1. Slice two limes and squeeze the juice into a bowl. Add the Lime essential oil.
2. Add 1 cup of Rose petals and the milk to the bowl. Mix well.
3. Pour mixture into running bathwater. Slice the third lime and add to the bath to float on top, along with the second cup of Rose petals.

FLOWER POWER MILK BATH

Enjoy this fragrant bouquet of Rose Geranium, Lavender and Orange for a sweet, relaxing feminine bath. The milk and Sweet Almond oil will add extra moisturizing benefits to the skin, leaving it feeling soft and silky.

What You Will Need:

9 drops Orange essential oil

1 drop Lavender essential oil

3 drops Rose Geranium essential oil

2 cups Powdered Milk

½ cup Cornstarch

¼ cup Baking Soda

2 teaspoon Sweet Almond oil

Bowl

What To Do:

1. In a bowl, combine all of the dry ingredients and Sweet Almond oil.
2. Add essential oils and mix well.
3. Pour the mixture into a flow of running water. Swish around to make sure the essential oils are evenly distributed.
4. Relax and soak in tub for 10-15 minutes.

ISLAND ESCAPE MILK BATH

What You Will Need:

4 ounces Powdered Milk

2 ounces Citric Acid

2 ounces Cornstarch

30 drops Grapefruit essential oil

60 drops Jasmine essential oil

What To Do:

1. Blend the powdered milk and cornstarch and sift.
2. Add the essential oils and citric acid. Stir well. Combine the citric acid mixture with the cornstarch blend.
3. To use, add 3 tablespoons to running bathwater.

BOHEMIAN MAMA MILK BATH

What You Will Need:

10 drops Bergamot essential oil

9 drops Orange essential oil

1 drop Rose Geranium essential oil

1 drop Ylang Ylang or Jasmine essential oil

2 drops Patchouli essential oil

2 teaspoon Sweet Almond oil

2 cups Powdered Milk

½ cup Cornstarch

¼ cup Baking Soda

What To Do:

1. In a bowl, blend dry ingredients together.
2. Add the Sweet Almond oil and essential oils. Mix well.
3. Pour the mixture into a warm bath of running water. Swish around to make sure the essential oils are evenly distributed.
4. Relax and soak in tub for 10-15 minutes.

Caution: Do not use this blend before sun exposure—it may increase the risk of sunburn.

SILK & SPICE MILK BATH

What You Will Need:

3 cups Powdered Milk

½ cup Cornstarch

¼ cup Baking Soda

10 drops Lavender essential oil

9 drops Patchouli or Sandalwood essential oil

1 drop Clove essential oil

2 teaspoons Sweet Almond oil

Bowl

What To Do:

1. In a bowl, blend all of the dry ingredients together.
2. Add Sweet Almond oil and essential oils. Mix well.
3. Pour the mixture into a warm bath of running water. Swish around to make sure the essential oils are evenly distributed.
4. Relax and soak in tub for 10-15 minutes.

Caution: If your skin is sensitive, leave out the Clove essential oil.

HEAVENLY VANILLA MILK BATH

What You Will Need:

10 drops Vanilla essential oil

2 teaspoons Sweet Almond oil

2 cups Powdered Milk

½ cup Cornstarch

¼ cup Baking Soda

Bowl

What To Do:

1. In a bowl, blend all of the dry ingredients together.
2. Add Sweet Almond oil and essential oils. Mix well.
3. Add the mixture to a warm bath of running water. Swish around to make sure the essential oils are evenly distributed.
4. Relax and soak in tub for 10-15 minutes.

SUMMER ROSE MILK BATH

What You Will Need:

6 drops Rose essential oil

3 drops Palmarosa essential oil

1 drop Rose Geranium essential oil

2 cups Powdered Milk

½ cup Cornstarch

¼ cup Baking Soda

2 teaspoons Sweet Almond oil

Bowl

What To Do:

1. In a bowl, blend all of the dry ingredients together.
2. Add Sweet Almond oil and essential oils. Mix well.
3. Add the mixture to a warm bath of running water. Swish around to make sure the essential oils are evenly distributed.
4. Relax and soak in tub for 10-15 minutes.

CUSTOM-SCENTED MILK BATH

What You Will Need:

1 cup Powdered Milk

5-10 drops Essential oil (your choice)

Small Sock

What To Do:

1. Fill a small sock with powdered milk and 5-10 drops of your favorite essential oil.
2. Hang sock over the faucet and allow warm water to run over it as it fills the tub. Enjoy!

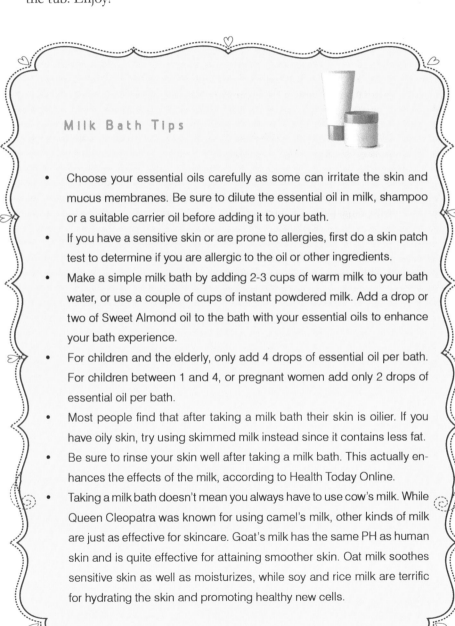

Milk Bath Tips

- Choose your essential oils carefully as some can irritate the skin and mucus membranes. Be sure to dilute the essential oil in milk, shampoo or a suitable carrier oil before adding it to your bath.
- If you have a sensitive skin or are prone to allergies, first do a skin patch test to determine if you are allergic to the oil or other ingredients.
- Make a simple milk bath by adding 2-3 cups of warm milk to your bath water, or use a couple of cups of instant powdered milk. Add a drop or two of Sweet Almond oil to the bath with your essential oils to enhance your bath experience.
- For children and the elderly, only add 4 drops of essential oil per bath. For children between 1 and 4, or pregnant women add only 2 drops of essential oil per bath.
- Most people find that after taking a milk bath their skin is oilier. If you have oily skin, try using skimmed milk instead since it contains less fat.
- Be sure to rinse your skin well after taking a milk bath. This actually enhances the effects of the milk, according to Health Today Online.
- Taking a milk bath doesn't mean you always have to use cow's milk. While Queen Cleopatra was known for using camel's milk, other kinds of milk are just as effective for skincare. Goat's milk has the same PH as human skin and is quite effective for attaining smoother skin. Oat milk soothes sensitive skin as well as moisturizes, while soy and rice milk are terrific for hydrating the skin and promoting healthy new cells.

Milk Bath Tips (continues)

- Find a pretty jar to store your premade powdered milk bath mix in, so it's always on hand ready for use.

- When you are ready to use your dry milk bath ingredients, stir in all the ingredients including the liquid components such as the water, honey and essential oils to make sure everything dissolves properly. Pour the mixture into your running bathwater and swish around. This way you will avoid the clumping of the dry materials along the sides of your bath and make clean up easier.

- Be sure to rinse the tub out carefully to make certain your bath doesn't stink or smell sour from the milk residue.

- The fragrant aroma of Mint opens up your senses, helping to rejuvenate your mind. Any mint will do—Peppermint, Spearmint, or Wintergreen.

- The tender fragrance of Rose in your bath will leave your skin supple and soft. Try adding fresh Rose petals to lift your spirits as they float across your skin. To make it even more romantic, add candles.

- Avoid using essential oils in the bath such as Oregano and Thyme and those with specific irritant potential such as Lemongrass. Phototoxic oils such as Bergamot should be used with caution.

- Essential oils that are generally regarded as safe and mild enough for the bath include: Lavender, Rose, Clary Sage, Geranium, Frankincense, Eucalyptus, Sandalwood, and conifers such as Cedarwood, Balsam Fir, Juniper, Pine, and Spruce to name a few.

Body Scrubs

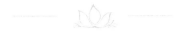

Essential oils can be incorporated into many facial products including scrubs and polishes. Exfoliating foot and body scrubs have become very popular and its no wonder—not only do they feel good to apply, but they also leave the skin feeling soft and wonderful afterwards! Try experimenting with different essential oils or blends and combining different exfoliating materials until you find your own personal favorite.

If the scrub will be used on children, the elderly, or pregnant, check with an Aromatherapist concerning the use of essential oils.

POMEGRANATE BODY SCRUB

What You Will Need:

½ cup Pomegranate seeds

½ cup White Unbleached Cane Sugar

2 teaspoons Pomegranate seed oil

1-2 drops Vanilla essential oil

Bowl

What To Do:

1. In a small bowl, mix the sugar and pomegranate seeds, crushing both with a spoon.
2. Add the essential oil and carrier oil and mix well.
3. Massage gently onto damp skin. Rinse off.

GINGER-MINT BODY SCRUB

Use this one in the morning to invigorate the body. Your skin will feel smoother and have a nice glow.

What You Will Need:

¼ cup Sea Salt

¼ cup Cornmeal

1/3 cup Olive oil

2 drops Ginger essential oil

4 drops Peppermint essential oil

3 drops Rosemary essential oil

What To Do:

Mix salt and cornmeal.

1. Warm the olive oil, and combine it with the essential oils. Mix with dry ingredients.
2. Use in the shower or standing in the tub. Apply in circular motions, working from the extremities inward, towards the center of the body and the heart. Rinse with warm water.

ORANGE-VANILLA BODY SCRUB

What You Will Need:

1 cup Epsom Salt

½ cup Olive oil

½ teaspoon Vanilla extract

4 drops Orange essential oil

What To Do:

1. In a small bowl, stir together all of the ingredients.
2. Place the scrub in small containers and give away as gifts or keep for yourself.

JUNIPER-LEMON THIGH SCRUB

This delightfully aromatic scrub works exfoliating wonders. The natural botanicals and cold-pressed oils work together to loosen stubborn cellulite and soften the surrounding skin. Massage your thighs twice a week for remarkable results.

What You Will Need:

1 small Avocado Stone

4 tablespoons Cornmeal

2 teaspoons Aloe Vera gel

1 tablespoon Grapeseed oil

6 drops Juniper essential oil

6 drops Lemon essential oil

What To Do:

1. Place the avocado pit in a heavy paper bag. With a hammer or wooden mallet, give the pit a few good whacks to break it up into smaller pieces that will fit into a coffee grinder or small food processor.
2. Grind the pieces to a gritty meal consistency. Mix in the cornmeal, place in a sterilized shallow jar and seal.
3. Pour the aloe, Grapeseed, Juniper, and Lemon essential oils into a bowl, then sprinkle about 2 teaspoons of the avocado and cornmeal over the wet ingredients and stir. Add additional meal if necessary so that you have a gritty paste.
4. Mist your legs thoroughly with body mist, then apply the paste, using small, circular, massaging motions. Relax for 15 minutes and rinse with warm water.

BROWN SUGAR LEG WAX

Most of us have seen the infomercials and the various leg sugaring products at the drugstore. It's so simple and inexpensive to make yourself, you'll always want to make your own!

What You Will Need:

2 cups Brown Sugar

4 drops Lemon essential oil

½ cup Water

2 tablespoons Glycerin

Waxing cloth strips or strips of linen

Wooden Popsicle sticks (to stir the wax and to apply)

What To Do:

1. Combine all of the ingredients in a saucepan. Stir frequently while heating to 250 degrees F.

2. Pour into jars and cover with lids.

To Use the Sugar Wax:

1. Heat in the microwave for 10 seconds on high. Using a wooden stick, stir very well. It should be warm but not hot. Please be very careful when heating up this wax—it's very easy to burn yourself. If the wax isn't warm enough, place it back in the microwave for 5 seconds, and stir again.

2. Lightly powder the area to be treated. Spread a thin layer of the wax on in the same direction as the hair grows.

3. Apply the waxing cloth strip over the applied wax, and rub down well to get the wax to stick to the cloth. Pull your skin taut, and in one quick motion pull the fabric off of your skin AGAINST the direction of hair growth.

4. Continue with the other areas of your leg or wherever you're waxing. When you're done waxing a complete area, rub in lotion, Aloe Vera gel (fresh is best), or oil to soothe your legs.

LAVENDER-ROSEMARY SALT SCRUB

This will give your skin a polished, moisturized glow while removing dull, dead cells.

What You Will Need:

1 ½ cup Sea Salt

½ cup Sweet Almond oil

1/8 cup Liquid Hand soap

5 capsules Vitamin E oil (or 12-15 drops)

½ teaspoon Peppermint essential oil

½ teaspoon Lavender essential oil

½ teaspoon Rosemary essential oil

Jar or container

What To Do:

1. Mix all of the ingredients in a jar or container. Stir well.
2. Add more salt if necessary or add more oil if too dry.
3. Shower as usual. Apply and then rinse off. Do not use on irritated skin or right after shaving.

GINGERBREAD MOLASSES BODY SCRUB

What You Will Need:

¾ cup Brown Sugar

1 teaspoon Freshly Grated Gingerroot

3 drops Ginger essential oil

1 teaspoon Cocoa Powder

1 tablespoon Molasses

What To Do:

1. In a bowl, add all of the ingredients and mix thoroughly.
2. To use, scoop up some of the scrub and rub it in circular motions all over your body.
3. Rinse well with warm water and pat skin dry with a towel.

OLIVE OIL BODY POLISH

What You Will Need:

1 cup Sea Salt, fine

½ cup Olive oil

½ cup Liquid Glycerin

½ teaspoon Peppermint essential oil

What To Do:

1. In a bowl, mix all of the ingredients together.

2. Store in a wide mouth jar. This scrub can be used on any part of the body.

GRAPEFRUIT SUGAR SCRUB

What You Will Need:

2/3 cup Granulated Sugar

1/3 cup Fine Salt

6-10 drops Grapefruit essential oil

Few drops Grapeseed oil (enough to make it scoopable)

What To Do:

1. Mix the sugar, salt, Grapeseed oil and Grapefruit essential oil to form a paste. Store in a jar.
2. While showering, invigorate your skin with the paste by rubbing on in circular motion all over the body.

FIELD & SEA BODY SCRUB

What You Will Need:

3 tablespoons Kelp powder

3 tablespoons Oatmeal

3 tablespoons Orange peel, grated

3 tablespoons Sea Salt

3 tablespoons Sunflower seeds, ground

3 drops Grapefruit essential oil

Sweet Almond oil

What To Do:

1. Mix all dry ingredients and Grapefruit essential oil in a jar. Keep jar sealed until ready to use.
2. Blend with Sweet Almond oil to the desired consistency just before using.

COFFEE BODY SCRUB

Use this for an invigorating scrub.

What You Will Need:

1 cup Ground Coffee

¾ cup Olive oil

½ cup Honey

2 drops Coffee essential oil

What To Do:

1. In a bowl, add all of the ingredients and mix together.
2. Use in the shower by scrubbing into the body using a washcloth or net scrubby. This will leave your skin silky smooth.

CREAMY CHOCOLATE BODY SCRUB

What You Will Need:

½ cup Raw Sugar

1/3 cup Cocoa

2 tablespoons Olive oil

2 drops Cacao absolute oil

What To Do:

1. In a bowl, combine all of the ingredients and mix thoroughly.
2. Apply the mixture to moistened skin and scrub with a facecloth or net scrubby.
3. Rinse thoroughly.

LEMON-LIME SALT SCRUB

What You Will Need:

2/3 cup Fine Sea Salt

1/3 cup Olive oil

1/3 cup Liquid Glycerin

1 zest Orange, grated

10 drops Orange essential oil

10 drops Lemon essential oil

10 drops Lime essential oil

What To Do:

1. In a glass bowl, mix the salt, olive oil, and soap.
2. Add the essential oil and orange zest. Stir well.
3. Transfer to a glass jar. Use as a body scrub when having a bath or a shower. Rinse off with warm water.

CUSTOM-SCENTED BODY SCRUB

This scrub is perfect after a bath or shower while the skin is still warm and damp.

What You Will Need:

1½ -2 cups Sea Salt, fine

¾ cup Olive oil

¾ cup Sweet Almond oil

12-15 drops Essential oils (your choice)

What To Do:

1. Mix salt, olive oil, and almond oil in a glass bowl.
2. Add an essential oil, such as Peppermint, for scent.
3. Store in a tightly sealed glass jar.
4. To use, massage a tablespoon or two onto the skin in small circles. Leave on for 5-20 minutes, then rinse.

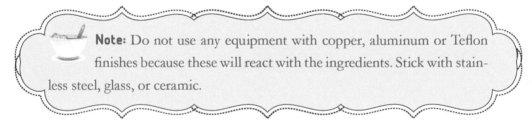

Note: Do not use any equipment with copper, aluminum or Teflon finishes because these will react with the ingredients. Stick with stainless steel, glass, or ceramic.

Bath Scrub Tips

- Use ultramarine powders or other natural powders and natural food coloring to color your scrubs.
- Try different coarsenesses of salt or sugar to create progressively smoother scrubs (for example, a coarse "buffing" scrub, followed by a fine "polishing" scrub) with different essential oils for each scrub.
- Spice things up by using brown sugar, table salt, or white sugar as your exfoliating agent instead of sea salt (or try combining two or more exfoliating agents) to get a different feel for your scrub.
- To polish up patchy remnants of a tan, take your Loofah into the bath with you and add several drops of Lemon essential oil or ¾ cup of Lemon juice to your bath to help bleach a fading tan and remove flaky skin. Or, add a few drops of Lemon essential oil to a sugar or salt paste and leave on skin for 30 minutes then rinse off.
- Try adding oatmeal to a bath to relieve sunburns. For exfoliating, fill an old sock with oatmeal then swish around in the bath water. After it has softened, scrub your body with it.
- Vinegar restores the acid balance of skin and also acts as a gentle exfoliate. Add 1 cup of raw apple cider vinegar to a lukewarm bath to ease itchy, peeling skin.
- There is a vast array of essential oils you can use in your body scrubs. Refer to the chapter, *Essential Oils for the Skin*, to determine which oils are best for your skin type.

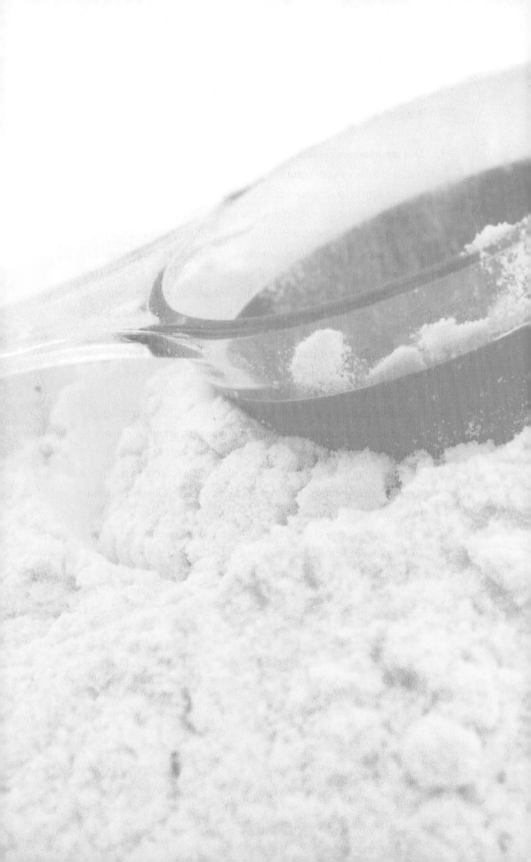

Body Powders

To add a soft, alluring scent to the body when a heavy perfume is overkill, dusting your body with a light homemade body powder is a great alternative. Dusting powder provides soothing relief for the skin that has been overexposed to heat and moisture as well as prevents further chafing, lessening irritation.

Making a natural body powder without the talc (which can contain asbestos) is really quite simple to do. You can even create medicated or foot powders economically at home. Most recipes consist only of a couple of ingredients: a base powder such as arrowroot or cornstarch and an essential oil or two. A few basic recipes are listed here, but the possible combinations of your favorite essential oil are endless. Just make sure the essential oil you choose is safe and beneficial for your skin.

LAVENDER BODY POWDER

This one is especially good for the feet!

What You Will Need:

1 cup Cornstarch

1 tablespoon Baking Soda

10-15 drops Lavender essential oil

2-5 drops Roman Chamomile essential oil

What To Do:

1. Mix the dry ingredients in a jar with a tight fitting lid.
2. Add the essential oils. Shake well.

WHITE BLOSSOMS DUSTING POWDER

What You Will Need:

¾ cup Arrowroot Powder

¼ cup Cornstarch

6 drops Honeysuckle essential oil

6 drops White Patchouli essential oil

What To Do:

1. In a bowl or with a mortar and pestle, mix all of the dry ingredients.
2. Add essential oils one drop at a time. Stir well.
3. If you have oily skin, you can substitute up to ½ ounce of white Kaolin powder for the Arrowroot powder, which will help absorb oil.

FAIRY DUST POWDER

What You Will Need:

½ cup Rice flour

½ cup Cornstarch

2 teaspoons Rose petals, finely crushed

½ teaspoon Mica

3 drops Rose essential oil

Shaker or container

What To Do:

1. In a bowl, mix all of the dry ingredients together.
2. Add the Rose essential oil. Stir well.
3. Store in an airtight container or shaker.

JASMINE BODY POWDER

What You Will Need:

1 cup Cornstarch

1 tablespoon Jasmine flowers, dried

1 teaspoon Sweet Almond oil

2 drops Jasmine essential oil

Shaker or container with lid

What To Do:

1. In a bowl, mix cornstarch, Jasmine flowers, and oils together. Stir well.

2. Place in an airtight container or shaker.

ARABIAN NIGHTS BATH POWDER

What You Will Need:

½ cup Baking Soda

½ cup Cornstarch or Arrowroot Powder

5 drops Patchouli essential oil

4 drops Sage essential oil

5 drops Sandalwood essential oil

Shaker or container with lid

What To Do:

1. In a bowl, combine all of the dry ingredients. Stir well.

2. Add the essential oils, one drop at a time. Blend thoroughly.

3. Store in a reusable container and enjoy!

SUGARY SPICE BATH POWDER

What You Will Need:

¾ cup Cornstarch

1 tablespoons Arrowroot Powder

5 drops Cassia or Cinnamon essential oil

¼ teaspoon Powdered Sugar

Shaker or container with lid

What To Do:

1. In a bowl, combine all of the dry ingredients. Stir well.

2. Add the essential oils, one drop at a time. Blend thoroughly.

3. Store in a reusable container and enjoy!

BODY ODOR DUSTING POWDER

What You Will Need:

4 ounces White Clay

8 drops Lavender essential oil

3 drops Coriander essential oil

Container with lid

What To Do:

1. In a container, add the clay and essential oils.
2. Replace lid and shake well. Used as needed.

CUSTOM-SCENTED BATH POWDER

What You Will Need:

½ cup Cornstarch

2 tablespoons Arrowroot Powder

2 tablespoons Baking Soda

10 drops Essential oil (your choice)

Shaker or container with lid

What To Do:

1. In a bowl, combine all of the dry ingredients and mix well.
2. Add the essential oils one drop at a time.
3. Let stand a few days to dry, and then sift through a flour sifter.
4. Pour into a powder shaker/container.

Bath Powder Tips

- Use only pure essential oils for your natural bath powders—not fragrance oil.
- Some of the most popular essential oils for your DIY body powders include: Lavender, Tea Tree, Peppermint, Jasmine, Rose, Sandalwood, Gardenia, Roman Chamomile, Comfrey, Marigold, and Neroli.
- A great way to store your bath powders is to use an old fashion sugar shaker. Look for old glass containers at yard sales, flea markets or antique shops. Or, recycle an old powder container from home and add a new puff from the dollar store. You can also visit a craft or beauty supply store for cosmetic supplies and glass jars.
- If the essential oil you choose causes skin irritation, rinse with cold water and discontinue use. If your skin is sensitive to the oils, fresh Rose petals or potpourri can be used in place of oils. It may take up to three days for these ingredients to scent the dry ingredients. Simply sift out the rose petals or herbs from the dry ingredients and use as you would a normal body powder.
- Besides dusting your body with powder after a bath or shower, you can also lightly sprinkle on bedding for a nicely scented sleep and scent lingerie drawers or closets. Scented powders make great homemade gifts.
- Make a homemade bath powder for your dog using Lavender or Tea Tree essential oil. Use between baths to help with odor.
- Have a favorite cologne you'd like to use as a bath powder? Place some cornstarch in a nice container and spritz your cologne or perfume into the container. Stir, cover and let set overnight.

Body Sprays and Mists

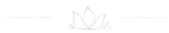

Fragrant essential oils can now go with you throughout the day in body sprays and mists. Just spray and go! And, making natural body sprays couldn't be easier!

Simply choose from your favorite aromatic essential oils that are safe for your skin and few other ingredients like distilled water or witch hazel and voila—you've created your own signature body mist! Body sprays are practically effortless to make with you in complete control over the ingredients you use, so you know what you are putting on your skin. For folks who suffer from allergies, this is a relief from commercial sprays full of artificial dyes and chemicals that can trigger adverse reactions.

Use these recipes as a starting point. Try different combinations of sweet-smelling essential oils, shake it up, and spray to test it until it finally suits you. You can even add a few drops of glycerin if you have it to make the spray last longer and act as a moisturizer. Feel free to be creative!

FALLING STARS BODY MIST

What You Will Need:

2 cups Distilled Water

3 tablespoons Organic Vodka

5 drops Lavender essential oil

10 drops Roman Chamomile essential oil

10 drops Valerian essential oil

What To Do:

1. Mix all of the ingredients together in a spray bottle and shake well.
2. Allow to settle for at least 12 hours. Store in a cool dry place.

AMAZE BODY MIST

What You Will Need:

2 cups Distilled Water

3 tablespoons Organic Vodka

5 drops St. John's Wort essential oil

10 drops Cypress essential oil

10 drops Rosemary essential oil

What To Do:

1. Mix all of the ingredients together in a spray bottle and shake well.
2. Allow to settle for at least 12 hours. Store in a cool dry place.

CITRUS BLOSSOMS BODY SPLASH

What You Will Need:

2 cups Distilled Water

3 tablespoons Organic Vodka

1 tablespoon Orange peel, finely chopped

1 tablespoon Lemon peel, finely chopped

5 drops Lemon Verbena essential oil

10 drops Mandarin essential oil

10 drops Orange essential oil

What To Do:

1. Combine the fruit peels with the vodka in a jar, cover and let stand for 1 week.
2. Strain the liquid and add the essential oils and water to the liquid.
3. Let stand for 2 weeks, shaking jar once a day. Keep in a dark bottle or keep in a cool dark area.

COOLING SUMMER BODY SPRAY

For a refreshingly cool spray, this recipe is great for use after showering.

What You Will Need:

1 tablespoon Witch Hazel

8 drops Lemon essential oil

2 drops Ginger essential oil

2 drops Peppermint essential oil

1 teaspoon Fresh Cucumber juice

1 cup Water

Spray bottle

What To Do:

1. Combine all of the ingredients in a spray bottle. Shake well.
2. To use, simply spritz onto skin.

SUNBURN HEALING SPRAY

Use this to cool down over-exposed skin from the sun's scorching rays!

What You Will Need:

½ cup Distilled Water

¼ cup Witch Hazel

½ cup Aloe Vera juice

8 drops Lavender essential oil

2 drops Roman Chamomile essential oil

1 drop Geranium essential oil

1 teaspoon Honey

Spray Bottle

What To Do:

1. In an 8-ounce spray bottle, add water, witch hazel and Aloe Vera juice.
2. In a small bowl, combine the essential oils and honey. Stir well to blend.
3. Pour the honey mixture into a bottle and shake to mix.
4. To use, spray on affected areas several times a day as needed.

ENCHANTED BODY MIST

What You Will Need:

2 cups Distilled Water

3 tablespoons Organic Vodka

5 drops Helichrysum essential oil

10 drops Peony essential oil

10 drops Sandalwood essential oil

What To Do:

1. Mix all of the ingredients together in a spray bottle and shake well.
2. Allow to settle for at least 12 hours. Store in a dry, cool place.

HERB GARDEN SPLASH

What You Will Need:

2 cups White Vinegar

¼ cup Honey

1 teaspoon Savory, dried

1 teaspoon Cloves, ground

1 teaspoon Bay leaves, crushed

2 drops Sage essential oil

2 drops Thyme essential oil

2 drops Clove essential oil

Glass jar or bottle

What To Do:

1. Combine all of the ingredients in a glass jar or container.
2. Store for 1 week, shaking occasionally to mix contents.
3. Strain and pour into a tightly capped bottle.

WHISPERING RAIN BODY MIST

What You Will Need:

2 cups Distilled Water

3 tablespoons Organic Vodka

5 drops Sandalwood essential oil

10 drops Bergamot essential oil

10 drops Cassia essential oil

Spray bottle

What To Do:

1. Mix all of the ingredients together in a spray bottle and shake well.
2. Allow to settle for at least 12 hours. Store in a cool dry place.

CUSTOM-SCENTED BODY SPRAY

What You Will Need:

2 cups Distilled Water

30-40 drops Essential oil (your choice)

Spray bottle

What To Do:

1. Mix all of the ingredients together in a spray bottle and shake well.
2. Allow to settle for at least 12 hours. Store in a cool dry place.

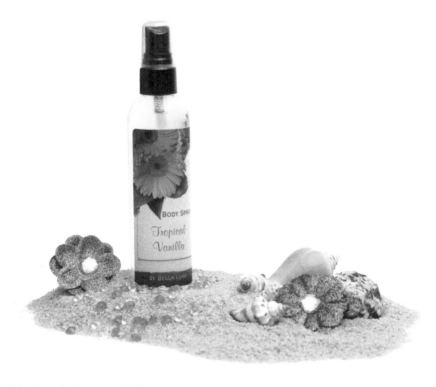

Body Spray & Mist Tips

- For creating simply delightful body sprays, try adding essential oils such as Orange, Lemon, Lime or Vanilla. These fragrances will help brighten your mood and those around you. These fragrances are effective for seasonal depression, especially during the dark, winter months.
- To add deodorizing benefits to your body sprays, use essential oils such as Bergamot, Eucalyptus, or Lemon.
- For a stimulating spray that will invigorate your senses and increasing mental activity include Peppermint and Grapefruit.
- For a more romantic scent, try using Rose and Ylang Ylang essential oils. These fragrances have been noted as having an aphrodisiac effect.
- For dog bedding, use Cedarwood or Tea Tree essential oils in a spray to spritz for flea control. Lemongrass essential oil is also good to calm over-excited pets and serve as an insect repellant.
- When making room sprays, try using calming oils such as Roman Chamomile or Lavender essential oils. Not only are these great as air fresheners, they enhance the atmosphere by promoting tranquility. These will also help promote restful sleep at night.
- Follow these simple guidelines for making facial mists, body sprays and room sprays:

  To make a facial mist, use 8-10 drops of essential oils per 4 ounces of distilled water.

  To make a body spray, use 30-40 drops of essential oils per 4 ounces of distilled water.

  To make a room spray, use 80-100 drops of essential oils per 4 ounces of distilled water.
- Purchase small pocketsize spray bottles from a dollar store or craft supply store. Fill with your favorite body spray and carry in your purse to use anytime!

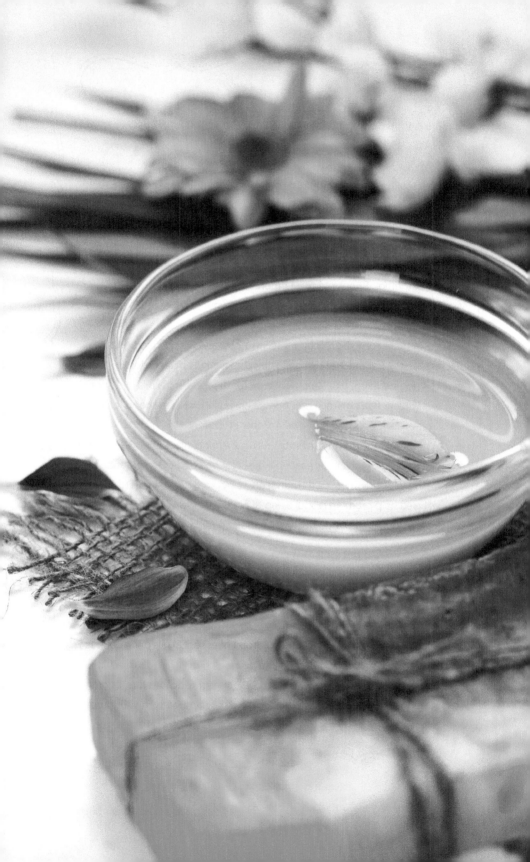

Body Lotions and Creams

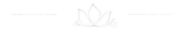

There are a variety of products on the market today that promise a more natural healthy look. Unfortunately, many of these products contain harmful chemicals and don't offer nature's best alternative to healthy-looking skin like essential oils do.

Making your own lotions and creams can really make a difference when therapeutic grade essential oils are included. Of course, don't expect results overnight. It will take time to see results as your skin regenerates, usually 28-37 days. So, be patient!

ORANGE-ALMOND BODY LOTION

Wrinkles, lines and sun damage have met their match! Try this lotion for its silky feel.

What You Will Need:

1/8 teaspoon Borax Powder

½ cup Sweet Almond oil

1 teaspoon Coconut oil

1 teaspoon Beeswax

2 tablespoons Honey

3-4 drops Orange essential oil

Jar or container

What To Do:

1. Combine all of the ingredients into a bowl. Stir to blend well.
2. Store in a jar or container until ready for use.

JASMINE BODY LOTION

What You Will Need:

¼ cup Apricot Kernel oil

1 teaspoon Beeswax

1 teaspoon Cocoa butter

1 teaspoon Coconut oil

¼ cup Distilled Water

1 teaspoon Aloe Vera gel

½ teaspoon Glycerin

5 drops Jasmine essential oil

What To Do:

1. Melt the cocoa butter, beeswax, apricot kernel oil and coconut oil over low heat. Allow to cool.
2. Measure the water, Aloe Vera gel and glycerin into a deep bowl.
3. Slowly drizzle in a small amount of the oil mixture and beat vigorously with a wire whisk. Continue to drizzle and beat until all the oil is blended into the water.
4. Stir in 5 drops of Jasmine essential oil.
5. Pour mixture into a container, label and enjoy.

CITRUS COOLER BODY LOTION

What You Will Need:

4 tablespoons Glycerin

40 drops Orange essential oil

4 tablespoons Lemon juice

What To Do:

1. Combine all of the ingredients in a clean glass bottle.
2. Shake well and refrigerate until ready to use.

OVERNIGHT BODY LOTION

This lush and creamy body lotion contains Lavender and Ylang Ylang, which will enrich your mind and body. It is extremely moisturizing and great for using before bed.

What You Will Need:

½ ounce Beeswax

½ ounce Cocoa butter

2 ounces Coconut oil

2 tablespoons Sweet Almond oil

4 tablespoons Mineral Water

½ teaspoon Lavender essential oil

½ teaspoon Ylang Ylang essential oil

Jar with lid

What To Do:

1. Slowly melt the sweet almond, beeswax, cocoa butter and coconut oil in a pan over low heat.
2. Use a whisk to beat the water in vigorously.
3. Remove the saucepan from the heat and continue stirring until the cream cools down.
4. Add the essential oils and blend well.
5. Stir until creamy. Pour into a jar with lid. Store in a dark, cool place to preserve the essential oils.

ROSE & GALBANUM BODY LOTION

Galbanum essential oil is effective for cell regeneration and when combined with Rose helps fight wrinkles and heal broken capillaries.

What You Will Need:

1/8 teaspoon Borax Powder

½ cup Sunflower oil

1 teaspoon Coconut oil

1 teaspoon Beeswax

½ cup Rosewater

5 drops Galbanum essential oil

4 drops Rose essential oil

Jar or container with lid

What To Do:

1. In a glass measuring cup, add the sunflower oil, coconut oil, and beeswax. Place the oil/beeswax mixture in a pan of water (about 1-2 inches of water), making a water bath.

2. Heat over medium heat until the beeswax is melted (8-10 minutes), stirring occasionally.

3. Mix the rosewater and the borax in a glass measuring cup. Place in the microwave on high for 1 minute.

4. Remove the oil/beeswax mixture from the water bath. Slowly add rosewater/borax to the mixture and whip in the blender.

5. Allow the lotion to cool completely. The consistency may seem a bit thin, but it will thicken as it cools.

6. Add the Galbanum and Rose essential oils.

7. Pour the lotion into a clean container with a lid. To use, massage a small amount into your skin.

LAVENDER LOTION

What You Will Need:

1 ounce Glycerin

2 teaspoons Lavender essential oil

What To Do:

1. Place the glycerin and Lavender essential oil in a clean glass bottle and shake well.

2. Refrigerate. Use as normal.

SUN-KISSED ORANGE LOTION

What You Will Need:

2 tablespoons Cocoa butter, melted

4 tablespoons Olive oil, warmed

4 tablespoons Orange juice

2 drops Orange essential oil

Bottle or Jar

What To Do:

1. Place all of the ingredients into a blender and mix until light and fluffy.
2. Store in a tightly capped bottle or jar. If the mixture separates, beat again.

ROSEMARY LOTION

What You Will Need:

2 ounces Rosewater

6 drops Rosemary essential oil

1 tablespoon Egg White

Jar with lid

What To Do:

1. Add all of the ingredients into a blender. Blend well.
2. Store in a clean, tightly capped jar in the refrigerator.

WOUND SKINCARE LOTION

What You Will Need:

10-12 drops Lavender essential oil

2-3 drops Helichrysum essential oil

5 drops Niaouli essential oil

2-3 drops Carrot Seed essential oil

½ tablespoon Calendula oil

½ tablespoon Rosehip Seed oil

1 capsule Vitamin E oil (or 2-3 drops)

Bottle

What To Do:

1. In a 1-ounce glass bottle, add carrier and essential oils. Shake to blend.

2. To use, pour a few drops on a clean wound. Cover with gauze.

MASSAGE LOTION BAR

What You Will Need:

½ cup Cocoa Butter, melted

10 capsules Vitamin E oil (or 25-30 drops)

1 tablespoon Coconut oil, melted

10 drops Rose essential oil

8 drops Peppermint essential oil

5 drops Ylang Ylang essential oil

Molds

What To Do:

1. In a pan, melt the cocoa butter, coconut oil, and vitamin E oil.

2. Let the mixture cool a bit then add the essential oils, one oil at a time. Blend well.

3. Pour into molds and let harden.

ECZEMA CREAM

What You Will Need:

8 ounces Un-Petroleum Jelly

4 ounces Beeswax

1 tablespoon Lanolin

10-15 drops Lavender essential oil

What To Do:

1. Place the beeswax in a double boiler. Add the un-petroleum jelly (see recipe at the end of this chapter) and lanolin. Melt over low heat, stirring constantly to combine ingredients.

2. Remove from heat and add the essential oil. Stir constantly until it thickens and cools.

3. Pour into glass jar or container until ready for use.

4. To use, rub a little dab into the affected area right after a bath while the skin is still moist (but not wet).

EXQUISITE REFRIGERATED LOTION BAR

This lotion bar is designed to literally melt into your skin, but not in your hands. It contains moisture rich cocoa butter, along with other luscious oils and butters that leave your skin feeling pampered and refined.

What You Will Need:

8 ounces Cocoa butter

1 ounce Shea butter

½ ounce Mango butter

½ ounce Avocado oil

1 teaspoon Calendula total CO2

2 teaspoons Liquid Grapefruit Seed extract

40 drops Essential oils (suggestions: Patchouli, Peppermint, Sandalwood, Lime, Rose or Vanilla)

What To Do:

1. Place the butters and avocado oil in a double boiler. (You could use a microwave to speed things up, but the extreme heat will all but destroy the nutrients in the oils if they are cold-pressed.)

2. Once the ingredients have melted, remove from heat. Stir with a clean wooden stir stick to ensure they are mixed. Allow to cool for about 15 minutes.

3. Add Grapefruit Seed extract and Calendula. Stir to blend well.

4. Add up to ¼ ounce of essential oils. Stir well.

5. Using a one-ounce candy tray or plastic mini muffin-sized tray, pour mixture in and place in the freezer for about 20 minutes.

6. When finished, gently release the bars from their mold and allow them to rest for a few hours before wrapping.

7. These bars are best stored in the refrigerator. They can be used in place of lotion. Give someone you love a special massage treat. Yields 10 luscious one-ounce bars.

PSORIASIS RELIEF CREAM

What You Will Need:

2 drops Patchouli essential oil

2 drops Roman Chamomile essential oil

2 drops Lavender essential oil

1 ounce Organic Unscented Body Lotion

What To Do:

1. In a bottle, add all the ingredients. Shake well to blend.
2. 2. Apply as needed to affected areas.

ROSE-GERANIUM FLORAL CREAM

What You Will Need:

¼ cup Distilled Water

½ teaspoon Borax Powder

3 tablespoons Beeswax

½ cup Mineral oil

1 teaspoon Lanolin

5 drops Rose essential oil

3 drops Geranium essential oil

What To Do:

1. Boil the water and add the Borax powder. Stir until dissolved.
2. Let this mixture simmer. In a separate heavy saucepan, add mineral oil, lanolin and beeswax, and place over low heat. Stir until the beeswax is dissolved.
3. Pour the oil/beeswax mixture into a bowl and slowly drizzle in the simmering water/borax mixture while stirring with a wire whisk. Continue

stirring until the mixture becomes a thick, white cream and has cooled to room temperature, approximately 15 minutes.

4. Stir in the essential oils until well blended. Spoon into a bottle or jar.

MILK & HONEY CLEANSING CREAM

What You Will Need:

1 teaspoon Honey

1 tablespoon Milk or Cream

4 drops Vanilla essential oil

What To Do:

1. Warm honey in the microwave or stovetop. Add milk or cream and essential oil.

2. Use as a cleanser while bathing or showering. This recipe should be prepared fresh each time.

JOJOBA-ALOE VERA MOISTURIZING CREAM

What You Will Need:

2 tablespoons Jojoba oil

1 tablespoon Beeswax

1 tablespoon Cocoa butter

1 tablespoon Vitamin E oil

4 tablespoons Aloe Vera gel

1 tablespoon Glycerin

20-30 drops Essential oil (your choice)

What To Do:

1. Heat the jojoba, beeswax, cocoa butter, and vitamin E oil in a double boiler at 160 degrees F.

2. Mix the aloe and glycerin in a second double boiler, also at 160 degrees F.

3. Remove both mixtures from the stove and slowly pour the oil mixture into the aloe/glycerin mixture while stirring.

4. Keep stirring until mixture cools then add essential oils and bottle. Makes about 4 ounces.

PEPPERMINT-WHEAT GERM STIMULATING CREAM

What You Will Need:

1 ounce Beeswax

3 ounces Wheat Germ oil

1 ounce Peppermint tea, brewed strong

1 drop Peppermint essential oil

Jar

What To Do:

1. Place all of the ingredients in a pan and heat on low until the beeswax is melted.

2. Remove from heat and whip with a whisk until cool.

3. Store in a glass jar until ready for use.

OUTDOOR LOTION

Use this lotion when attending outdoor events for protection without the insect repellant scent.

What You Will Need:

2 teaspoons Castor oil

1 teaspoon Lanolin

1 ½ teaspoon Cocoa butter

2 capsules Vitamin E oil (or 5-6 drops)

5 drops Lavender essential oil

3 drops Tea Tree essential oil

What To Do:

1. Melt the castor oil, lanolin and cocoa butter in a double boiler. Remove from heat.

2. Whisk the vitamin E oil into the mixture.

3. As it cools, add the essential oils, mixing well. Store in a bottle or jar.

INSECT REPELLANT CREAM

What You Will Need:

¼ cup Pennyroyal-infused Grapeseed oil

¼ cup Olive oil

1 teaspoon Coconut oil

2 tablespoons Beeswax

1/8 teaspoon Borax Powder

¼ cup Distilled Water

5 drops Lemongrass essential oil

3 drops Citronella essential oil

20 drops Lavender essential oil

10 drops Rosemary essential oil

10 drops Eucalyptus essential oil

10 drops Pine needle essential oil

20 drops Cedarwood essential oil

What To Do:

1. Melt together the pennyroyal-infused oil, beeswax, olive and coconut oil.
2. While wax is melting, pour the distilled water and borax in a pint jelly jar, and microwave for less than a minute to dissolve borax.
3. When beeswax is melted, pour oil/wax mixture into the borax/water mixture and stir to blend.
4. Add each essential oil one at a time, stirring to mix well.
5. Replace lid on the jelly jar and shake vigorously, until mixture starts to become a cream (it will not take long). Makes 1 pint.

BUG OFF LOTION BAR

Use these bars on a camping trip or when you're going on a hike in the woods!

What You Will Need:

4 ounces Beeswax

4 ounces Shea Butter

3 ounces Avocado oil

1 ounce Grapeseed oil

½ teaspoon Eucalyptus essential oil

½ teaspoon Citronella essential oil

½ teaspoon Lemongrass essential oil

What To Do:

1. In a double boiler, melt the beeswax and Shea butter. When it is completely melted, add the avocado and Grapeseed oils. Mix well.
2. Pour into a bowl and allow to cool slightly.
3. Add the essential oils, one at a time, and stir to blend.
4. Pour mixture into molds. Let it sit for several hours.

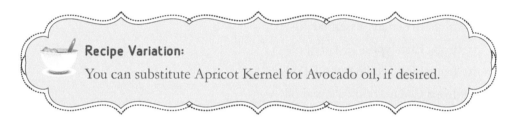

Recipe Variation:

You can substitute Apricot Kernel for Avocado oil, if desired.

OLIVE OIL SHAVING CREAM

What You Will Need:

¼ cup Stearic Acid

2 tablespoons Olive Oil

1 cup Hot Water

1 teaspoon Borax Powder

2 tablespoons Soap, grated

What To Do:

1. Melt the Stearic acid and oil in double boiler until clear liquid forms.
2. In another container, add hot water, borax, and soap, stirring until the borax and soap are dissolved. Pour the soap solution into a blender and blend well for about 1 minute.
3. Slowly pour the melted Stearic acid mixture into the soap solution. Blend on high until a smooth cream forms.
4. Pour into a clean container and allow to cool completely.

5. To use, splash warm water on legs then apply the shaving cream. Use a sharp, clean razor.

STICK DEODORANT

What You Will Need:

4 ounces Cornstarch

2 ounces Baking Soda

1 ounce Liquid chlorophyll

2 ounces Organic Vodka

2 ounces Distilled Water

8 ounces Beeswax

10-15 drops Coriander essential oil

What To Do:
1. Mix all of the ingredients except the wax, chlorophyll, and essential oil in a bowl, stirring thoroughly.
2. Melt the wax in a double boiler over very low heat then remove from heat.
3. Add to the mixed ingredients and blend well. If the wax thickens too much to be workable, heat again.
4. As the mixture begins to cool, but before it hardens, add the liquid chlorophyll and essential oil. Pour into molds and let harden.
5. Store in a tightly closed container away from heat to avoid shrinkage.

UN-PETROLEUM JELLY (HOMEMADE VASELINE)

What You Will Need:

1 ounce Beeswax

½ cup Olive Oil

Essential Oil (optional)

Jar

What To Do:
1. In a saucepan, mix the ingredients together on low heat until the beeswax has melted.

2. Add several drops of essential oil, if desired.

3. Pour into a jar or container while it is still warm.

4. Use in place of Vaseline. You can also use in recipes that call for un-petroleum jelly.

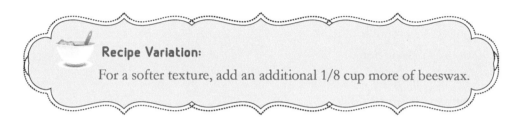

Recipe Variation:

For a softer texture, add an additional 1/8 cup more of beeswax.

CUSTOM-SCENTED BODY LOTION

What You Will Need:

1 cup Distilled Water

¾ cup carrier oil (such as Olive, Almond, Unrefined Coconut, or Avocado)

3 tablespoons Beeswax, grated

12 drops Essential oils (your choice)

Blender

Saucepan

Jars

What To Do:

1. Place the carrier oils and beeswax in a glass measuring cup. Place the cup in a water bath making sure the water reaches about halfway up the cup.

2. Bring the water to a gentle boil and heat until the beeswax melts. Remove the cup from the water and let the mixture cool for 2 minutes.

3. Pour the water into the blender and run at medium speed. Slowly add the beeswax/oil mixture while running (through the blender stopper lid) until it begins to emulsify.

4. Add your essential oils and blend.

5. Transfer the cream to a glass jar. Cover the jar with cheesecloth for an hour, or until it has reached room temperature.

6. Place the lid on each jar after the lotion has cooled completely. It can be stored at room temperature for up to 3 months or in the refrigerator for 6 months.

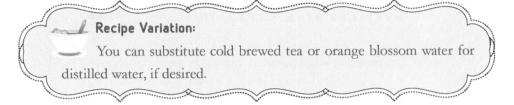

Recipe Variation:
You can substitute cold brewed tea or orange blossom water for distilled water, if desired.

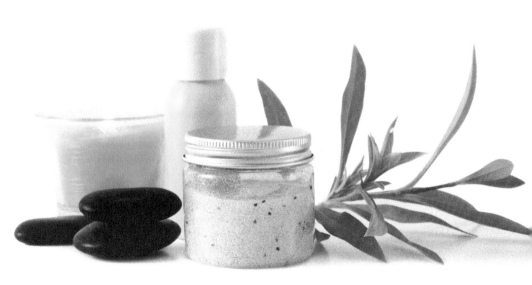

Body Lotion & Cream Tips

- When treating a skin condition, make sure the essential oil you choose is safe for your skin. If this is the first time using essential oils in a body lotion or cream, be sure to do a skin patch test to check for any allergic reaction.

- Try experimenting with different essential oils for different therapeutic effects.

- The essential oils of Lavender, Geranium, Neroli, Rosemary, Rose, and Frankincense are historic "anti-aging" ingredients for mature skin. Jasmine, Myrrh, Carrot Seed, and Helichrysum also rejuvenate the skin, encouraging new cell growth.

- Set aside an old blender, a small glass bowl, and a spatula solely for making your natural aromatherapy products since beeswax found in creams and lotions can leave a residue on the blender and utensils used.

- Ingredients like extracts and botanicals can reduce the shelf life of your product dramatically, and need to be well preserved. Before adding any ingredient, know the shelf life and how it can affect your end product.

- Adding Vitamin E oil to your products can extend the shelf life!

- Experiment by replacing the water called for in a recipe with floral water such as orange blossom or an herbal infusion. You can also add color to your lotions by using brew pink hibiscus tea or green tea in place of water.

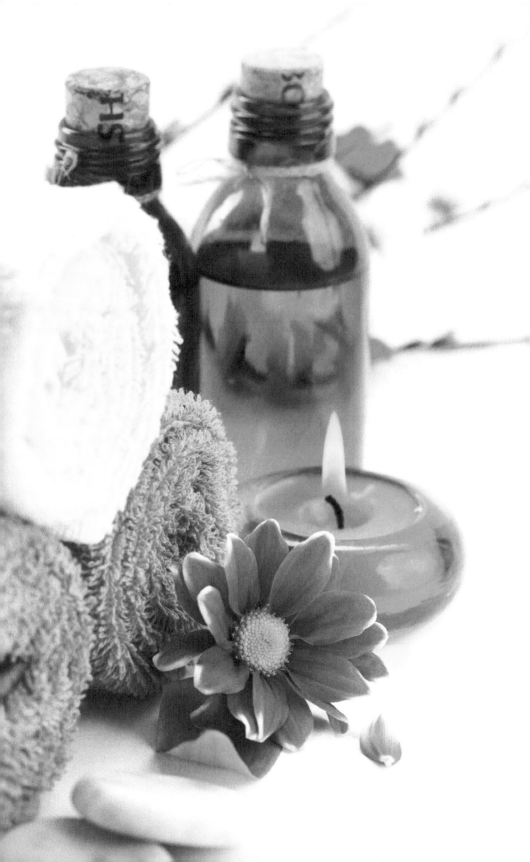

Massage Oils

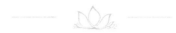

There are a endless variety of massage styles to choose from—almost as many as there are massage oil recipes! Your selection of an appropriate massage oil recipe to make and use will depend upon which style of massage you have in mind. While massage oils are used primarily for lubrication, the essential oils and carrier oil used in your blend can offer many healthy benefits for the skin and the body.

Soothing achy muscles with a massage oil consisting of essential oils not only stimulates the circulation of blood, delivering healing to the body's soft tissues, but its aroma can be very comforting, calming the mind.

For a more relaxing or sensual massage, the most important consideration will be your personal choice. The massage oil recipe you choose can certainly enhance this very plea-surable "scentual" experience. But, if the person giving or receiving the massage does not find the blend of oils agreeable, it could also spoil the moment. Spend time getting familiar with the various essential oil scents to help guide you in finding those blends that are most appealing.

When selecting an oil blend for your massage, here are some things to consider:

- Style of massage
- Skin type of the receiver, i.e. dry, oily, mature, or sensitive
- Purpose of the massage, i.e. relaxation or sore muscle relief
- Aromatic preferences of the receiver
- Sensitivities or allergies

This chapter includes many massage oil recipes to choose from. Massage oils are very open to personal interpretation and the addition or deletion of essential oils and carrier oils can be adjusted to your personal preference.

Once you have selected a massage oil recipe to use, add each essential oil one at a time to a dark, glass bottle. Next, add the carrier oil. Replace the bottle's lid and shake to mix.

To use, warm up the blend by rolling the bottle between the palms of your hands prior to doing a massage. Always be sure to test essential oils for skin sensitivity before using any product directly on your skin.

Make Your Own Sensuous Massage Oil

If you prefer experimenting, why not try creating your own blend. It's easy!

First, choose three or four different essential oils for your blend, depending on the effect or benefit you are hoping to achieve such as Clary Sage, Geranium, Grapefruit, Jasmine absolute, Mandarin, Myrrh, Neroli, Orange, Patchouli, Petitgrain, Rose, Sandalwood, Vanilla, Vetiver, or Ylang Ylang.

In a dark colored glass bottle, add 15-30 drops of your essential oils. As a general rule, you can use up to 15 drops of essential oil per 1 ounce of carrier oil. It is always better to start with fewer drops of essential oils and add more later, if necessary.

Next, choose a carrier oil such as Jojoba, Grapeseed, Fractionated Coconut, Rosehip, Olive, Macadamia Nut, Sesame Seed, or Sweet Almond. Pour 1 ounce of the vegetable oil into a small glass bottle (1 ounce equals 1/8 cup, 2 tablespoons, or approximately 30 milliliters). Gently shake the bottle to mix the oils.

Create a label with the massage oil name, what the ingredients are, and how to use it. For example, your label might read: "Peace and Love Massage Oil contains: Jojoba oil and natural essential oils of Patchouli and Sandalwood. Apply to desired area and massage oil into the skin."

Massage oils make wonderful personalized gifts for weddings, anniversaries, birthdays, or any other special occasion. Give a single bottle, or create a massage gift-pack with several varieties of oils.

Try this: At Home "Hot Stone" Spa Treatment

Find a large, flat, smooth stone that fits nicely in the palm of your hand. Wash thoroughly then heat in a pan of water or in the oven until it is warm, not hot. Rub one of your scented massage oil blends onto the stone and use on partner for a soothing massage. The heat from the stone along with the essential oils will relax and penetrate muscles.

SENSUAL MASSAGE OIL

½ cup Fractionated Coconut oil
3 drops Rose essential oil
3 drops Lavender essential oil

PEACE & LOVE MASSAGE OIL

1 ounce Jojoba oil
3 drops Patchouli essential oil
3 drops Sandalwood essential oil

ROMANTIC MASSAGE OIL

1 ounce Sweet Almond oil
6 drops Lavender essential oil
4 drops Orange essential oil
3 drops Ylang Ylang essential oil
2 drops Clary Sage essential oil

EXOTIC MASSAGE OIL

1 ounce Sweet Almond oil
7 drops Ylang Ylang essential oil
6 drops Geranium essential oil
5 drops Sandalwood essential oil

4 drops Patchouli essential oil
3 drops Clary Sage essential oil

WILD FIELDS MASSAGE OIL

1 ounce Grapeseed oil
6 drops Roman Chamomile essential oil
2 drops Rose essential oil
2 drops Rosemary essential oil

BLOSSOM GROVE MASSAGE OIL

8 teaspoons Grapeseed oil
6 drops Orange essential oil
2 drops Lemongrass essential oil
2 drops Neroli essential oil

CRESCENT MOON MASSAGE OIL

10 teaspoons Wheat Germ oil
6 drops Roman Chamomile essential oil
4 drops Neroli essential oil
2 drops Rose essential oil
1 drop Basil essential oil

DREAM TOUCH MASSAGE OIL

¼ cup Fractionated Coconut oil
4 drops Clary Sage essential oil
3 drops Ylang Ylang essential oil
5 drops Neroli essential oil

ARABIAN NIGHTS EROTIC MASSAGE OIL

1 ounce Sweet Almond oil

3 drops Coriander essential oil

3 drops Frankincense essential oil

2 drops Lime essential oil

2 drops Rose essential oil

EXOTIC PATCHOULI MASSAGE OIL

10 teaspoons Grapeseed oil

7 drops Patchouli essential oil

4 drops Jasmine essential oil

2 drops Rose essential oil

SULTRY NIGHTS EROTIC MASSAGE OIL

1 ounce Sweet Almond oil

3 drops Geranium essential oil

2 drops Patchouli essential oil

3 drops Rose essential oil

EXQUISITE SANDALWOOD MASSAGE OIL

10 teaspoons Grapeseed oil

6 drops Sandalwood essential oil

2 drops Lavender essential oil

2 drops Rosewood essential oil

2 drops Rose essential oil

FALL HARVEST MASSAGE OIL

2 ounces Grapeseed oil

6 drops Bergamot essential oil

2 drops Cardamom essential oil

2 drops Jasmine essential oil

1 drop Orange essential oil

FOREST NIGHTS MASSAGE OIL

10 teaspoons Grapeseed oil

5 drops Rosewood essential oil

2 drops Cedarwood essential oil

2 drops German Chamomile essential oil

OLD SPICE MANLY MASSAGE OIL

¼ cup Jojoba oil

¼ cup Sweet Almond oil

6 drops Sandalwood essential oil

4 drops Bay essential oil

3 drops Bergamot essential oil

2 drops Lime essential oil

MINTY FRESH MASSAGE OIL

½ ounce Sweet Almond oil

3 drops Eucalyptus essential oil

4 drops Rosemary essential oil

2 drops Peppermint essential oil

NIGHT DREAMS MASSAGE OIL

10 teaspoons Grapeseed oil

6 drops Roman Chamomile essential oil

4 drops Jasmine essential oil

2 drops Rose essential oil

1 drop Lavender essential oil

ORIENTAL DELIGHT MASSAGE OIL

8 teaspoons Peanut oil

6 drops Orange essential oil

2 drops Sandalwood essential oil

2 drops Rosemary essential oil

1 drop Jasmine essential oil

PASSAGE OF INDIA MASSAGE OIL

10 teaspoons Grapeseed oil

7 drops Sandalwood essential oil

2 drops Orange essential oil

2 drops Rose essential oil

1 drop Cinnamon essential oil

FLOWERY ESCAPE MASSAGE OIL

1 ounce Grapeseed oil

7 drops Rosewood essential oil

4 drops Geranium essential oil

4 drops Jasmine essential oil

SPICY MASSAGE OIL

1 ounce Fractionated Coconut oil

7 drops Sandalwood essential oil

4 drops Cinnamon essential oil

3 drops Peppermint essential oil

2 drops Black Pepper essential oil

STIMULATING MASSAGE OIL

1 ounce Sweet Almond oil

5 drops Rose essential oil

7 drops Ylang Ylang essential oil

3 drops Jasmine essential oil

SEDUCTION MASSAGE OIL

½ ounce Jojoba oil

2 drops Cardamom essential oil

4 drops Ginger essential oil

5 drops Patchouli essential oil

4 drops Sandalwood essential oil

MAGNETISM APHRODISIAC MASSAGE OIL

½ ounce Jojoba oil

3 drops Jasmine essential oil

3 drops Sandalwood essential oil

4 drops Tangerine essential oil

5 drops Ylang Ylang essential oil

INVIGORATING MASSAGE OIL

½ ounce Sweet Almond oil

½ ounce Grapeseed oil

½ ounce Apricot Kernel oil

5 drops Lemon essential oil

5 drops Bergamot essential oil

5 drops Eucalyptus essential oil

5 drops Lavender essential oil

FEELING FRISKY MASSAGE OIL

½ ounce Jojoba oil

1 drop Jasmine essential oil

2 drops Grapefruit essential oil

3 drops Sandalwood essential oil

4 drops Bergamot essential oil

REFRESHING MASSAGE OIL

½ ounce Jojoba oil

4 drops Bergamot essential oil

2 drops Grapefruit essential oil

2 drops Ylang Ylang essential oil

2 drops Lemon essential oil

ENERGIZING MASSAGE OIL

1 ounce Sweet Almond oil

11 drops Lemon essential oil

6 drops Bergamot essential oil

3 drops Spearmint essential oil

REVIVING MASSAGE OIL

1 ounce Jojoba oil

4 drops Clary Sage essential oil

4 drops Ylang Ylang essential oil

2 drops Bergamot essential oil

PRIMAL MASSAGE OIL

3 teaspoons Grapeseed oil

2 drops Grapefruit essential oil

2 drops Basil essential oil

1 drop Cypress essential oil

GOOD MORNING MASSAGE OIL

3 teaspoons Sweet Almond oil

3 drops Grapefruit essential oil

2 drops Ginger essential oil

VITALIZING MASSAGE OIL

3 teaspoons Fractionated Coconut oil

3 drops Bergamot essential oil

2 drops Rosemary essential oil

BRISK MASSAGE OIL

1 ounce Fractionated Coconut oil

2 drops Lemon essential oil

2 drops Peppermint essential oil

1 drop Frankincense essential oil

SOOTHING SENSATIONS MASSAGE OIL

10 teaspoons Safflower oil

5 drops Lavender essential oil

2 drops Violet essential oil

2 drops Roman Chamomile essential oil

2 drops Frankincense essential oil

SPICE OF LIFE MASSAGE OIL

10 teaspoons Olive oil

6 drops Ginger essential oil

4 drops Jasmine essential oil

2 drops Orange essential oil

TEMPTATIONS MASSAGE OIL

1 ounce Grapeseed oil

6 drops Jasmine essential oil

2 drops Tea Tree essential oil

2 drops Neroli essential oil

RED ROSE LOVE MASSAGE OIL

½ ounce Grapeseed oil

1 drop Rose essential oil

2 drops Grapefruit essential oil

2 drops Ylang Ylang essential oil

MOON MAGIC MASSAGE OIL

½ ounce Sweet Almond oil

1 drop Coriander essential oil

2 drops Sandalwood essential oil

2 drops Lemon essential oil

2 drops Ylang Ylang essential oil

WINTER NIGHTS WARMING MASSAGE OIL

1 ounce Sweet Almond oil

10 drops Vanilla essential oil

5 drops Basil essential oil

COCONUT LIME TROPICAL MASSAGE OIL

2 ounces Macadamia Nut oil

2 ounces Fractionated Coconut oil

2 ounces Jojoba oil

1 ounce Rosehip oil

15 drops Lime essential oil

10 drops Vanilla essential oil

5 drops Coconut essential oil

SCENTSATIONAL MASSAGE OIL

1 ounce Sunflower oil

½ ounce Rosehip oil

½ ounce Jojoba oil

10 drops Tangerine essential oil

10 drops Sandalwood essential oil

10 drops Ylang Ylang essential oil

PMS MASSAGE OIL

1 ounce Fractionated Coconut oil

2 drops Carrot Seed essential oil

3 drops Clary Sage essential oil

3 drops Fennel essential oil

5 drops Lavender essential oil

8 drops Marjoram essential oil

2 drops Mugwort essential oil

5 drops Rosewood essential oil

POSTPARTUM DEPRESSION MASSAGE OIL

2 tablespoons Rosehip Seed oil

8 drops Geranium essential oil

10 drops Grapefruit essential oil

6 drops Mandarin essential oil

4 drops Neroli essential oil

PRE-MENSTRUAL MASSAGE OIL

2 ounces Fractionated Coconut oil

10 drops Geranium essential oil

15 drops Lavender essential oil

5 drops German Chamomile essential oil

3 drops Cypress essential oil

STRETCH MARKS MASSAGE OIL

4 drops Rose essential oil

1 drop Rosemary essential oil

4 drops Lavender essential oil

4 drops Neroli essential oil

1 drop Geranium essential oil

½ teaspoon Camellia oil

½ teaspoon Sesame oil

½ teaspoon Vitamin E oil

½ teaspoon Wheat Germ oil

TROUBLE SPOTS MASSAGE OIL

2 tablespoons Jojoba oil

10 drops Lavender essential oil

8 drops Rosemary essential oil

4 drops Ginger essential oil

3 drops Peppermint essential oil

HOT FLASHES MASSAGE OIL

2 tablespoons Almond oil

10 drops Grapefruit essential oil

10 drops Lime essential oil

7 drops Sage essential oil

3 drops Thyme essential oil

HORMONAL HEADACHE MASSAGE OIL

1 ounce Fractionated Coconut oil

2 drops Roman Chamomile essential oil

2 drops German Chamomile essential oil

4 drops Geranium essential oil

2 drops Myrtle essential oil

1 drop Nutmeg essential oil

3 drops Sage essential oil

1 drop Spearmint essential oil

ANTI-CELLULITE MASSAGE OIL

2 tablespoons Sweet Almond oil

5 drops Carrot Seed essential oil

5 drops Jojoba oil

8 drops Fennel essential oil

14 drops Grapefruit essential oil

8 drops Lemon essential oil

DIURETIC MASSAGE OIL

1 ounce Fractionated Coconut oil

10 drops Fennel essential oil

12 drops Grapefruit essential oil

8 drops Juniper essential oil

DYSMENORRHEA MASSAGE OIL

2 ounces Evening Primrose oil

5 drops Roman Chamomile essential oil

5 drops German Chamomile essential oil

5 drops Clary Sage essential oil

5 drops Fennel essential oil

3 drops Marjoram essential oil

5 drops Mugwort essential oil

12 drops Lavender essential oil

EXHAUSTION MASSAGE OIL

1 ounce Jojoba oil

5 drops Coriander essential oil

5 drops Grapefruit essential oil

5 drops Lavender essential oil

FAT ATTACK MASSAGE OIL

1 ounce and 2 tablespoons Sweet Almond oil

8 drops Cypress essential oil

5 drops Grapefruit essential oil

2 drops Oregano essential oil

5 drops Rosemary essential oil

5 drops Carrot Seed essential oil

SORE RELIEF MASSAGE OIL

½ ounce Olive oil

5 drops Rosemary essential oil

3 drops German Chamomile essential oil

2 drops Lavender essential oil

3 drops Marjoram essential oil

MUSCULAR TENSION MASSAGE OIL

1 ounce Sunflower oil

½ ounce Rosehip Seed oil

½ ounce Jojoba oil

10 drops Rosemary essential oil

10 drops Lavender essential oil

10 drops Marjoram essential oil

ACHY MUSCLE MASSAGE OIL

1 ounce Sweet Almond oil

2 drops Ginger essential oil

4 drops Peppermint essential oil

5 drops Eucalyptus essential oil

1 drop Black Pepper essential oil

COOL DOWN MASSAGE OIL

1 ounce Sweet Almond oil

10 drops Pine essential oil

2 drops Sandalwood essential oil

2 drops Clary Sage essential oil

LAVENDER CALMING MASSAGE OIL

1 ounce Sweet Almond oil

1 ounce Sunflower oil

2 ounces Grapeseed oil

1 ounce Apricot Kernel oil

15 drops Lavender essential oil

5 drops Frankincense essential oil

DE-STRESS MASSAGE OIL

1 ounce Sweet Almond oil

6 drops Clary Sage essential oil

2 drops Lemon essential oil

3 drops Lavender essential oil

4 drops Roman Chamomile essential oil

ANTI-WRINKLE MASSAGE OIL

1 ounce Rosehip oil

2 drops Rose essential oil

1 drop Rosemary essential oil

2 drops Rosewood essential oil

3 drops Sandalwood essential oil

CUSTOM-SCENTED MASSAGE OIL

1 ounce Carrier oil (your choice)

8 drops Essential oil (your choice)

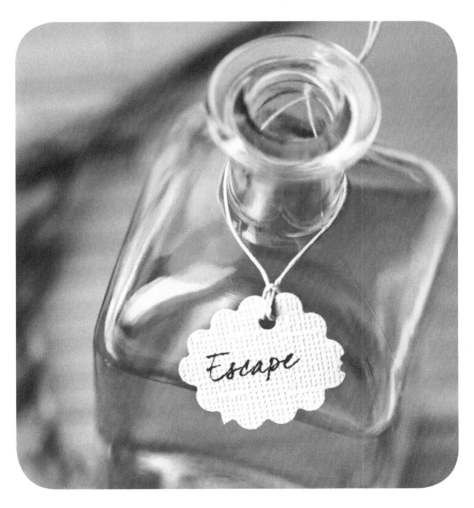

Massage Oil Tips

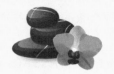

- Your massage oil blend can be used in other ways as well. Here are some suggestions

- Feel free to substitute any of the carrier oils called for in a recipe to give it a different feel or fragrance.

- Dab on 1-2 drops undiluted (without carrier oil) as a perfume.

- Add 3 drops undiluted to a room diffuser, light ring, or candle.

- Add 6 drops into a running bath of warm water.

- Use 5 drops in a bowl of hot water for a foot bath.

- Dab a few drops of your massage oil blend undiluted on a tissue or cotton ball and gently wave in the air as a room freshener.

- Blow out a lit candle then add a few drops of your massage oil blend undiluted to the melted wax. Relight the candle for a wonderful room perfume.

- Essential oils for a calming or relaxing massage oil may include: Roman Chamomile, Cedarwood, Lavender, Clary Sage, Jasmine, Frankincense, Patchouli, Ylang Ylang, or Sandalwood.

- Essential oils that help create an invigorating and energizing massage oil could include: Basil, Bergamot, Black Pepper, Cypress, Rosemary, Lime, or Eucalyptus.

- Essential oils that create a romantic massage oil may include: Aloes, Sandalwood, Cumin, Clove, Rose, Jasmine, Orange, Rosewood, Vanilla, or Ylang Ylang.

- Author Margie Hare in her book, "Aromatherapy Massage," suggests using Lavender or Geranium essential oils for normal skin, Patchouli or Rosewood for dry skin, Lemon or Cypress for oily skin, and Sandalwood or Chamomile for sensitive skin. For more information on which oils to use for your particular skin condition, refer to the chapter, *Essential Oils for the Skin*.

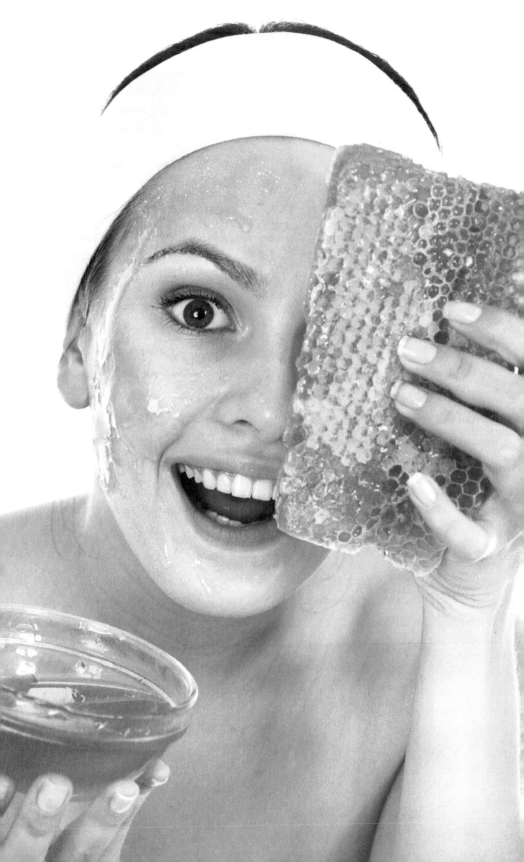

Essential Care for the Face

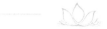

Caring for your face is a delicate matter and should be one of your highest priorities. While many of us simply splash water and go, years of neglect soon catch up with signs of premature aging from overexposure to the sun's UV rays and other environmental toxins. By adding essential oils to your daily beauty regimen you will be able to diminish wrinkles and receive many other benefits from the oils such as their powerful antioxidant, antiseptic, anti-fungal, and anti-bacterial qualities. In addition, essential oils used in facial products have the unique and superior advantage over synthetic products in their capacity to advance cellular renewal by increasing circulation and hydration. The recipes for facial treatments in this section contain ingredients that not only help nourish the skin and allow it to maintain its own natural beauty but will also boost your immunity, reduce stress, and balance emotions—all of which factor into maintaining healthy, young-looking skin.

Each person is unique, and what may work for one person may not be the best formula for another. Other things may factor in, such as diet, exercise, and lifestyle. Try different combinations and experiment with the oils. If a recipe doesn't work for you, you may only need to tweak it by substituting one essential oil. Once you get a few recipes that work for you, it is good to keep alternating recipes from day to day, or week to week, to allow your face to get the benefit of other oils as well. Just like our body, our skin benefits from a variety of nutrients that are found in multiple sources.

Six Steps to Facial Care

Dead skin cells, perspiration, and grime from the atmosphere can clog your pores, giving your skin a dull and lifeless appearance. Here's a regimen that takes only minutes a day and will breathe life back in your complexion in no time flat.

As you select skin care recipes from this book that match your skin type, performing this simple regimen will produce almost immediate, visible results. If you already have a routine you may develop a more specific routine that suits you by adding these steps.

STEP ONE: STEAM. Before going to bed, soak a washcloth in steamy, hot water and wring lightly. Hold close to your face for 2 minutes. The steam will open your pores.

STEP TWO: CLEANSE. While your pores are open, splash warm water on your face and neck. Pour a workable amount of facial cleanser into your hands and rub together until it lathers. Using your fingertips (or facial brush), delicately massage into your skin in a circular motion for about 30 seconds. Avoid using harsh hand soap.

STEP THREE: EXFOLIATE. To ensure a radiant complexion, you will want to exfoliate to remove dead cells and encourage new cell growth, giving your skin that healthy glow. Be sure to use a delicate scrub. You'll find recipes in the chapter called, *Facial Scrubs.* Or, you may want to try a facial mask instead. It's a marvelous tool to keep your skin looking beautiful. You'll find those recipes in a chapter called, *Masks and Facials.* Indulge and enjoy!

Even though you're using natural homemade ingredients, treat your skin gently. Just because we call them "facial scrubs" doesn't mean you should scrub your skin the way you do the kitchen floor! If you treat your skin gently, you'll decrease the odds of damaging it and acquiring wrinkles.

STEP FOUR: TONE. Using a cotton ball, dampen with alcohol-free toner and gently wipe your entire face and neck.

STEP FIVE: MOISTURIZE. Your skin is craving it. Apply a small amount of moisturizer into your hands and work into your skin in an upward, circular motion. In order for moisturizer to work and protect your skin, it needs to be applied to a clean face! Many skin care experts recommend using moisturizers at night, so they can penetrate your skin undisturbed.

STEP SIX: APPLY OILS. After you have washed your face, leave it slightly damp. Apply 2-3 drops of your facial oil blend (20 drops of essential oils + 2 tablespoons of carrier oil) by lightly dabbing on to spread the oil in an upward motion. For dry and mature skin, you may want to add your essential oil to a light facial cream instead of carrier oil. For sunburned skin, use Aloe Vera gel as your carrier.

Remember to drink plenty of water. Keeping your skin hydrated goes a long way toward maintaining healthy skin. You've already been told that it improves the functioning of all of your cells and your organs—your skin is your largest organ, so this makes sense! Most health experts say to drink a minimum of 8-10 glasses of water a day. If you can do this, then you're doing your skin a big favor!

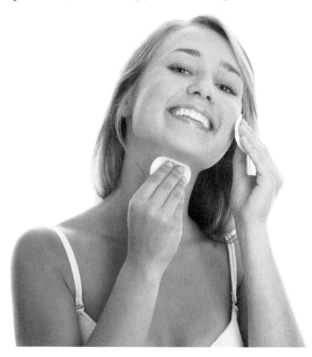

Facial Scrubs

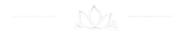

Facial scrubs are the next best thing to sliced bread when it comes to leaving your skin squeaky clean. If you haven't tried one yet, these are extremely easy to make and usually only require a few ingredients found in your kitchen such as oatmeal or cornmeal, almonds, honey, and yogurt.

HONEY WHEAT FACIAL SCRUB

What You Will Need:

2 tablespoons Bee Pollen

½ cup Honey

1 tablespoon Liquid Lecithin

¼ cup Almonds, ground

¼ cup Walnuts, ground

¼ cup Oatmeal

¼ cup Whole Wheat Flour

¼ cup Cornmeal

10-12 drops Orange essential oil

1 tablespoon Rosewater

¼ cup Water

What To Do:

1. Combine all of the dry ingredients.
2. Add the honey, Rosewater, essential oil and liquid lecithin to the dry ingredients.

3. Stir until smooth. Add enough water to make a smooth paste. Makes about 2 cups.
4. To use, wet face. Add 1 teaspoon of the scrub to your palm, moisten with water, and apply to face. Massage in a circular motion over face and neck. Leave on for 15 minutes. Rinse off with warm water. Use as a regular face wash or as needed to exfoliate.

LEMON-LIME FACIAL SCRUB

Great for your hands and feet too!

What You Will Need:

½ cup Sugar or Salt

1 tablespoon Olive oil

2 drops Lemon essential oil (or Lemon juice)

2 drops Lime essential oil

What To Do:

1. In a small bowl, mix all of the ingredients.
2. Pour into a pretty jar with a plastic spoon.
3. Use 1 tablespoon to scrub face, or add 2-3 tablespoons to bath water.

PATCHOULI-GRAPEFRUIT FACIAL SCRUB

What You Will Need:

¼ cup Yogurt

¼ cup Cornmeal

5 drops Patchouli essential oil

5 drops Grapefruit essential oil

What To Do:

1. Mix all of the ingredients together and refrigerate a couple of hours before using.
2. Store in the refrigerator until ready for use.

YOGURT-WALNUT FACIAL SCRUB

Walnuts make this scrub good for exfoliating while the yogurt and Lavender essential oil soothes the skin. Good for sensitive or irritated skin.

What You Will Need:

¼ cup Plain Yogurt

¼ cup Walnuts, ground

5 drops Lavender essential oil

What To Do:

1. Mix all of the ingredients together and refrigerate a couple of hours before using.
2. Store in the refrigerator until ready for use.

OATMEAL-ALMOND EXFOLIATING FACIAL SCRUB

What You Will Need:

½ cup Almonds, raw

½ cup Oatmeal, ground

10-12 drops Roman Chamomile essential oil

What To Do:

1. Grind almonds to a fine texture in a food processor or grinder.
2. Add ground oatmeal and essential oil. Mix well.
3. To use, wet face. Add 1 teaspoon of the scrub to your palm, moisten with water, and apply to face. Massage in a circular motion over face and neck. Rinse well with cool water. Use as a regular face wash or as needed to exfoliate.

SOOTHING STRAWBERRY-BANANA SCRUB

Use this scrub for normal or combination skin types. It's okay to lick your fingers with this one!

What You Will Need:

¼ cup Plain Yogurt

1 tablespoon Powdered Milk

3-4 pieces Strawberries, mashed

¼ Banana, mashed

2-3 drops Lemon essential oil

What To Do:

1. Mix all of the ingredients together and refrigerate a couple of hours before using.

2. Store in the refrigerator until ready for use.

3. To use, wet face. Apply directly to your face. Gently massage in a circular motion over face and neck. Rinse well with cool water and pat dry.

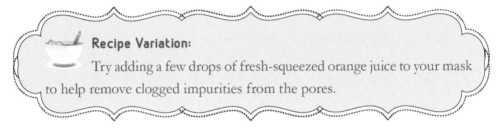

Recipe Variation:

Try adding a few drops of fresh-squeezed orange juice to your mask to help remove clogged impurities from the pores.

RAW SUGAR SCRUB

Don't be tempted to eat this one! It exfoliates dead skin cells from your face, leaving your skin incredibly soft.

What You Will Need:

1 cup Raw Sugar

1 cup Avocado oil (or substitute Glycerin)

Small amount Aloe Vera gel

2 drops Lavender essential oil

2 drops Orange essential oil

Mixing bowl

What To Do:

1. In a large mixing bowl, combine all ingredients.

2. Scoop some of the sugar scrub into your hands and massage gently onto your skin for 1 minute. You will begin to feel your skin tighten like a mask.

3. Leave on for 5 minutes before rinsing. You can use this on other parts of your body as well.

4. Some redness or blotches may develop after cleansing your skin. This is normal because of the deep cleaning.

DEEP CLEANSING CAT LITTER FACIAL SCRUB

This recipe calls for 100% natural, unscented cat litter—which is made from Bentonite clay. Bentonite clay helps to purge toxins and other impurities trapped within the pores.

What You Will Need:

4 tablespoons Cat litter, unscented

1 small Lemon, juice

Warm Water

2-3 drops Lemon essential oil

What To Do:

1. In a bowl, add the cat litter and the juice squeezed from one lemon.

2. Add water a little at a time and stir to make a paste.

3. Add essential oil and blend well.

4. To use, wet face. Add 1 teaspoon of the scrub to your palm, moisten with water, and apply to face. Massage in a circular motion over face and neck. Leave on for 15 minutes. Rinse off with warm water. Use as a regular face wash or as needed to exfoliate.

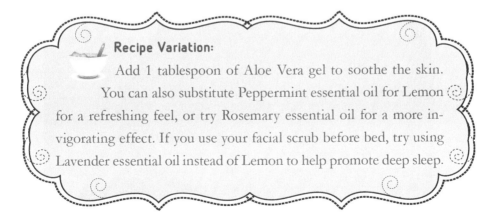

Recipe Variation:

Add 1 tablespoon of Aloe Vera gel to soothe the skin. You can also substitute Peppermint essential oil for Lemon for a refreshing feel, or try Rosemary essential oil for a more invigorating effect. If you use your facial scrub before bed, try using Lavender essential oil instead of Lemon to help promote deep sleep.

ROSEWOOD EXFOLIATING FACIAL SCRUB

This scrub works wonders by exfoliating dead skin leaving a soft finish!

What You Will Need:

2 tablespoons Raw Sugar

2 tablespoons Warm Water

2 drops Rosewood essential oil

What To Do:

1. In a small bowl, slowly add water to sugar until dissolved.
2. Add essential oil and stir well.
3. To use, apply to a clean face and gently massage into skin for 5 minutes. Rinse off with warm water. Pat dry.

CUSTOM-SCENTED FACIAL SCRUB

What You Will Need:

½ cup Fractionated Coconut oil (or another carrier oil)

1 cup Sugar or Salt (or another gritty substance)

4-5 drops Essential oil (your choice)

What To Do:

1. Pour the sugar or salt into a jar or bowl.
2. Add coconut oil and essential oils. Mix all of the ingredients well.
3. Use 1 tablespoon to scrub face, or add 2-3 tablespoons to bath water.

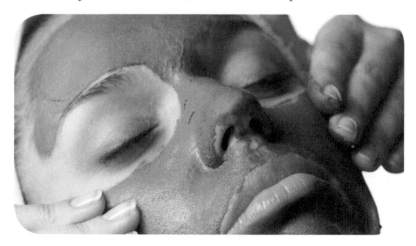

Facial Scrub Tips

- Be sure to cleanse your face thoroughly with a mild liquid cleanser before applying any facial mask or scrub.
- Choose an appropriate scrub with the best essential oils for your skin type. Do not use a scrub if you have extra sensitive skin.
- Take care not to use a scrub when you have angry looking pimples on your face. At times a scrub can aggravate the situation.
- Apply your scrub in an upward motion on the face. Be careful around the lips and sensitive areas, using only a couple fingers to apply.
- Use a facial brush with soft bristles to scrub the skin in a circular motion to slough away dead cells. This will help stimulate the blood's circulation in your face giving your complexion a warm glow. If you don't have a facial brush, massage the scrub into your face and neck using your fingertips.
- Use a soft moist towel or cleansing pad to remove the facial scrub, again gently rubbing skin in an upward motion. Rinse well to remove all of the scrub so that your skin will feel smooth and soft.
- Gently pat your skin dry with a soft towel and continue with the rest of your skin care regimen.
- Store your facial scrub container near your shower or tub (unless it requires refrigeration). That way you won't forget to use it, and in doing so, you will maintain your glow.
- Only use a facial scrub as often as is appropriate for your skin type. Some experts recommend only once a week. If you use it everyday, you will damage your skin, making it dry and dull.

Masks and Facials

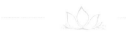

No need to spend a fortune on spa treatments and products when you can do your own masks and facials at home for pennies. Using simple ingredients found in the kitchen along with a few drops of essential oils, you can do more for your skin than just deep clean. Facial masks especially designed for your skin type can exfoliate, rejuvenate, nourish and hydrate your skin.

If you have acne-prone or oily skin, a clay-based mask works great for removing excess oils and impurities from deep within pores. They are especially good for preventing blackheads and balancing out your complexion.

For those with dry skin, a mask made with honey and oils help by nourishing your dehydrated skin. Red Clay is great for soothing sensitive skin.

Of course, all masks do not have to be clay-based. You can use honey, yogurt, oatmeal, whipped egg whites, or fruit as your base. Here are some other mask ingredients you may want to experiment with:

HONEY MASKS are great for exfoliating, hydrating and nourishing the skin, with mild antibacterial action while softening, soothing and healing. According to the National Honey board, honey naturally contains a "wide array of vitamins and minerals, including niacin, riboflavin, pantothenic acid, calcium, copper, iron, magnesium, manganese, phosphorus, potassium and zinc."

YOGURT AND CREAM MASKS not only exfoliate and nourish the skin, but help to restore the skin's acid balance; yogurt has a natural antibacterial action while the cream is moisturizing.

JUICES such as Lemon juice diluted with water (50/50) removes oil and gently bleaches freckles. Tomato juice is excellent for oily skin. Lettuce juice and pulp soothes sore, rough skin and heals blemishes. Pineapple juice works as an astringent and wash for oily skin. Orange juice hydrates mature skin, while watermelon juice gently exfoliates, softens and deep-cleanses.

WHIPPED EGG WHITES are excellent as an astringent, drying oily skin and for tightening pores and lifting sagging skin; simply whisk two egg whites and leave on your face for 10 minutes for an instant lift. For dry skin, try egg yokes.

MASHED FRUIT such as strawberries have fruit acids that exfoliate, cleanse and brighten skin, while also delivering anti-aging antioxidant action to your skin's surface. Other fruits such as bananas are nourishing, while pears help soothe hot sunburn, and apples are slightly acidic, soothing and gently exfoliating. Mashed apricots cleanse and moisturize the skin; cucumbers cool the skin, and are mild healers slightly bleaching freckles. Grapes are filled with alpha-hydroxy acids—an ingredient found in many skin firming and anti-wrinkle creams.

MASHED VEGGIES such as avocados is a highly nourishing mask rich in skin-friendly vitamins A, B and protein that deeply penetrates the skin. Other vegetables such as pumpkins and asparagus stimulate circulation and help dry up pimples, while carrot's pulp works as an antiseptic and heals pimples. Grated raw potato helps clear blemishes and eczema. Cooked and mashed turnips make a great deep-cleanser, as well as fresh fig pulp. Celery juice acts as a toner for older skin.

For pulped ingredients, blend enough raw ingredients with a little added water to make a tablespoon of pulp. Alternatively, you can boil raw vegetables in water then mash to make pulp.

While it is perfectly fine to use the raw pulp alone as a mask, adding a "binder" such as oatmeal, corn flour, ground almonds, or rolled oats will help hold it together better while adding healthy benefits good for your skin.

GRAINS such as oatmeal deeply cleanse while soothing irritated, inflamed or sensitive skin; sufferers of eczema can benefit from a weekly oatmeal mask. Cornmeal and other flours can be used as well.

BREWER'S YEAST is superb for oily skin. It contains all B group vitamins which are indispensable, especially inositol, folic acid and choline.

CLAY POWDERS such as Rose, White, or Bentonite are great for improving the skin. Mineral clays naturally absorb oil and dirt, cleansing pores and providing a deep clean; green clay is particularly beneficial for oily skin, drawing out oil while tightening pores. Red clay is great for sensitive and dry skin. White clay, the mildest of all the clays, works well on those with mature skin who desire it anti-aging properties and want to increase circulation.

DRIED MILK POWDER will both clean and moisturize your face wonderfully; very soothing and gentle.

GROUNDED NUTS, SEEDS AND BEANS all add a light exfoliating effect to your masks and make your skin glow.

Other foods good to use in masks include: apple cider vinegar, baking soda, brown sugar, cinnamon, butter, coffee (fine ground/brewed), tea (herbal and green) and fresh herbs from your kitchen windowsill garden.

Once you have selected base ingredients for your mask, simply add a tablespoon to a binder with 2-3 drops of essential oils that suit your skin type. After applying to skin, wait 20 minutes then rinse.

Skin Type Aromatherapy Masks

DRY OR DEHYDRATED SKIN Use a half mashed avocado as your base and add 2 drops of Patchouli essential oil and 1 drop of Sandalwood essential oil.

MATURE SKIN Use a thick cream or yogurt as your base and add 3 drops of vitamin A-rich Carrot Seed essential oil.

SENSITIVE SKIN Use ground oatmeal as your base then add 2 drops of Neroli essential oil.

OILY OR PROBLEM SKIN Use Green Kaolin clay as your base then add 2 drops of Cedarwood essential oil and 1 drop of Juniper essential oil.

MASK FOR NORMAL SKIN

This facial mask is a wonderful way to even out your skin's tone and make it glow.

What You Will Need:

2 tablespoons Green or Rose Clay

1 teaspoon Honey

2 drops Geranium essential oil

Aloe Vera juice

Bowl

What To Do:

1. In a bowl, add clay, honey and aloe juice.
2. Add essential oil one drop at a time. Stir well.
3. To use, apply to a slightly damp face. Leave on for 10-15 minutes. Rinse off with warm water. Pat skin dry.

MASK FOR DRY SKIN

What You Will Need:

1 tablespoon Rose Clay

1 tablespoon Instant Oatmeal or finely ground Regular Oatmeal

1 teaspoon Honey

1 teaspoon Sweet Almond oil

1 drop Rose essential oil

1 drop Lavender essential oil

Bowl

What To Do:

1. Add clay, oatmeal, honey and almond oil to a bowl and mix.
2. Add essential oils, one drop at a time. Stir well.
3. Stir in enough water to make a paste. If it is too runny, add more clay or oatmeal.

MASK FOR OILY SKIN

What You Will Need:

2 tablespoons Green Clay

1 teaspoon Aloe Vera juice

½ teaspoon Olive oil or Jojoba oil

1 drop Bergamot essential oil

1 drop Lavender essential oil

Bowl

What To Do:

1. Add clay, aloe juice and oil to the bowl and mix.
2. Add essential oils, one drop at a time. Stir well.
3. Stir in enough water to make a paste. If it is too runny, add a little more clay.
4. To use, apply to a slightly damp face. Leave on for 10-15 minutes. Rinse off with warm water. Pat skin dry.

MASK FOR SENSITIVE SKIN

What You Will Need:

1 tablespoon Rose Clay

1-2 teaspoons Avocado oil

1 drop Rose essential oil

1 drop Roman Chamomile essential oil

What To Do:

1. In a bowl, add clay and avocado oil.
2. Add essential oils. Stir well.
3. Use water, if necessary, to make a paste. Add more clay if it is too runny.

4. To use, apply to a slightly damp face. Leave on for 10-15 minutes. Rinse off with warm water. Pat skin dry.

MASK FOR MATURE / AGING SKIN

What You Will Need:

1 tablespoon Rose Clay

1 tablespoon Instant Oatmeal or finely ground Regular Oatmeal

1 teaspoon Honey

1 teaspoon Avocado or Sweet Almond oil

1 drop Frankincense essential oil

1 drop Neroli or Lavender essential oil

1 drop Rose essential oil

Water

Bowl

What To Do:

1. In a bowl, add clay, oatmeal, honey and oils.
2. Add enough water to make a soft paste. Massage into skin. Rinse well.

STRAWBERRIES & CREAM FACIAL MASK

Moisturize your skin weekly with this facial mask!

What You Will Need:

4-6 Ripe Strawberries

2 teaspoons Heavy Cream

1 teaspoon Honey

2-3 drops Niaouli essential oil

What To Do:

1. In a blender, puree the strawberries with the cream, essential oil and honey.
2. Apply to your face and leave on for 10 minutes. Rinse off with cool water. Pat skin dry.

BREWER'S YEAST FACIAL MASK

This facial mask is great for those with oily or combination skin types!

What You Will Need:

2 tablespoons Yogurt

1 teaspoon Brewer's Yeast

2-3 drops Spikenard essential oil

What To Do:

1. In a bowl, mix all of the ingredients. Stir well.
2. To use, apply facial mask to the T-zone (oily places on the face only). Wait for 10-15 minutes then rinse with warm water. Pat skin dry.

PEAS & CARROTS FACIAL MASK

When your mother told you to eat all your veggies, she must have known they would help protect your skin from premature wrinkles. This mask is great for normal and oily skin types.

What You Will Need:

¼ cup Peas, cooked and mashed

2-3 Carrots, cooked and mashed

4 ½ tablespoons Honey

1 drop Black Pepper essential oil

2 drops Parsley essential oil

What To Do:

1. In a bowl, add cooked peas and carrots and mash.
2. Add honey and essential oils. Stir well.
3. To use, apply facial mask to a clean face. Do not massage into skin. Leave on for 5-10 minutes then wash off with warm water. Pat dry.

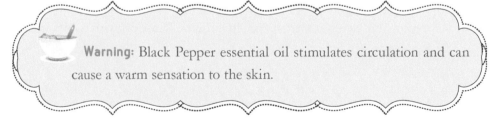

Warning: Black Pepper essential oil stimulates circulation and can cause a warm sensation to the skin.

EGG YOLK & HONEY FACIAL MASK

Use this facial to moisturize dry skin.

What You Will Need:

1 Egg Yolk

1 teaspoon Honey

1 teaspoon Whole Milk or Cream

2 drops Myrrh essential oil

What To Do:

1. In a bowl, mix all of the ingredients together.
2. To use, apply mask to face and leave on for 15-20 minutes.
3. Rinse off with warm water. Pat dry.

Recipe Variation:

If you are lactose intolerant, substitute 1 teaspoon of Olive oil for milk.

EGG WHITES & LEMON FACIAL MASK

What You Will Need:

1 tablespoon Oatmeal

2 Egg Whites (or Powdered Egg Whites)

2-3 drops Lemon essential oil

Bowl

What To Do:

1. In a small bowl, add oatmeal and egg whites (or powdered eggs).
2. Add essential oils and mix well.
3. Spread on face. Leave on until dry or 15-20 minutes. Rinse.

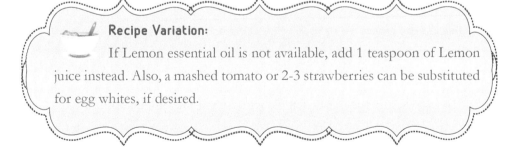

Recipe Variation:

   If Lemon essential oil is not available, add 1 teaspoon of Lemon juice instead. Also, a mashed tomato or 2-3 strawberries can be substituted for egg whites, if desired.

APRICOT & CREAM FACIAL MASK

This healing mask revitalizes the skin!

What You Will Need:

½ cup Dried Apricots, chopped

½ cup Warm Water

1 tablespoon Powdered Creamer (or Dry Milk Powder)

1 tablespoon Honey

2-3 drops Palmarosa essential oil

What To Do:

Add all of the ingredients into a blender and puree until smooth.

To use, apply to face and leave on for 15-20 minutes. Rinse off with warm water. Pat skin dry.

Recipe Variation:

For one of the most non-abrasive masks, try using Papaya instead of Apricots. Papaya is known to contain a strong enzyme called Papain which dissolves oil and dead skin cells.

APPLE & HONEY FACIAL MASK

Here's an easy treatment for acne or oily skin! Apples exfoliate the skin gently by removing dead skin cells with their natural extracts such as alpha hydroxyl acid. In addition, they protects the skin from bacteria and further acne breakouts.

What You Will Need:

1 Fresh Apple, mashed

5 tablespoons Honey

2 drops Helichrysum essential oil

What To Do:

1. In a bowl, mix the mashed apple with honey and essential oil.

2. Apply to the face immediately and leave on the face for 10 minutes. Rinse off with warm water. Pat skin dry.

POTATO & TOMATO FACIAL MASK

This mask is your secret weapon for cleansing oily skin and preventing future breakouts.

What You Will Need:

1 Tomato

2 tablespoons Potato flour

1-2 drops Basil essential oil

What To Do:

1. Peel the tomato and remove seeds.
2. In a bowl, mash tomato and add essential oil.
3. Add potato flour and stir until it forms a paste.
4. To use, apply to your face and leave on 15 minutes. Rinse off with warm water. Pat skin dry.

TURMERIC FACIAL MASK

Turmeric is known to slow down the aging process by stimulating the blood flow, which helps your skin stay healthy and retard the formation of wrinkles.

What You Will Need:

1 tablespoon Milk Powder

1 teaspoon Turmeric

1-2 drops Sandalwood essential oil

Several drops of Water

What To Do:

1. In a small bowl, combine the milk powder, turmeric, and essential oil. Add a few drops of water at a time while stirring until you have a smooth paste.
2. Apply to the face using your fingertips. Leave on for 10-15 minutes or until your skin feels tight and dry. Rinse off with cold water. Pat dry.

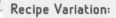
GRAPEFRUIT FACIAL MASK

What You Will Need:

1 teaspoon Sour Cream

1 Egg White

1 teaspoon Grapefruit juice

2-3 drops Grapefruit essential oil

What To Do:

1. In a bowl, beat an egg white until it is fluffy.
2. Add sour cream, essential oil, and juice. Stir well.
3. To use, apply to the face for 15 minutes. Rinse with warm water. Pat skin dry.

AVOCADO & CARROT FACIAL MASK

This moisturizing mask cleanses while leaving your skin smooth.

What You Will Need:

½ Avocado, ripe

1 Carrot

2-5 drops Carrot Seed essential oil

1 tablespoon Olive oil

Water

Pot

What To Do:

1. In a pot of water, boil the carrot until soft.

2. Place the carrot, avocado, essential oil and olive oil in a blender. Blend until it forms a paste.

3. To use, apply to your face and leave on for 20 minutes. Wash off with warm water. Pat skin dry.

YOGURT & BENTONITE CLAY MASK

What You Will Need:

1 teaspoon Hot Water

½ teaspoon Dead Sea Salt

2 teaspoons Buttermilk

2 tablespoons Plain Yogurt

5 drops German Chamomile essential oil

5 drops Lavender essential oil

3 drops Tea Tree essential oil

2 heaping tablespoons Bentonite Clay, powdered

Bowl

What To Do:

1. In a bowl, add buttermilk, yogurt, and clay.

2. Dissolve sea salts in hot water and stir in.

3. Add essential oils and blend well.

4. Spread on face and body. Leave on until dry or 20 minutes. Rinse with warm water. Pat skin dry.

SWAMP QUEEN FACIAL MASK

If you have an oily complexion, use this recipe for a deep cleansing once a week for a month.

What You Will Need:

3 tablespoons Green Clay (substitute White or Pink clays if you have sensitive or dry skin)

¼ cup Sweet Almond Oil

2 drops Rosemary essential oil

2 drops Lemon essential oil

2 drops Lavender essential oil

2 drops Geranium essential oil

2 slices Fresh Cucumber, peeled

2 small bowls

What To Do:

1. Be sure to clean your face thoroughly with a mild liquid cleanser before applying a facial mask.

2. In a bowl, combine green clay, Rosemary and Lemon essential oils. Apply clay mixture evenly on face and neck.

3. Place a cucumber slice over each eye. Lie back and relax for 10 minutes.

4. Rinse with warm water. Pat skin dry.

5. In another bowl, mix the carrier oil, Geranium and Lavender essential oils. For the finishing touch, apply to face for shine and moisturizing. Your face will glow!

FIRMING PEACH FACIAL

What You Will Need:

1 Ripe Peach

1 Egg White

1 teaspoon Yogurt

2 drops Myrtle essential oil

What To Do:

1. In a blender, puree all of the ingredients.

2. To use, apply to the face and leave on for 10-15 minutes to tighten sagging skin. Rinse off with warm water. Pat dry.

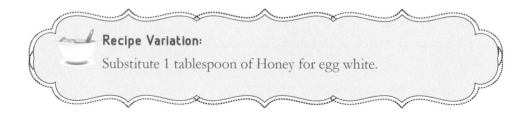

Recipe Variation:

Substitute 1 tablespoon of Honey for egg white.

LEMONGRASS & GERANIUM SKIN FACIAL

This facial is good for oily or combination skin types.

What You Will Need:

1 tablespoon Cornmeal

2 Eggs

2 drops Lemongrass essential oil

2 drops Geranium essential oil

What To Do:

1. Cleanse your face, steam, and splash with cool water. Pat skin dry.
2. Massage with the dry cornmeal. Rinse off.
3. Whip the eggs and add essential oils.
4. Brush on face. Leave on for 20 minutes then rinse off.

SUMMER SUN SOOTHER FACIAL

When you have been out in the sun too long, try using this refreshing mask to help heal sunburn!

What You Will Need:

½ cup Yogurt

¼ cup Oatmeal, grounded

2 drops Jasmine essential oil

What To Do:

1. In a bowl, mix all of the ingredients. Stir well.
2. To use, apply to over-exposed areas and leave on skin for 10 minutes. Rinse off with cool water. Pat dry.

CUCUMBER-YOGURT FACIAL

This is probably one of the most popular facial masks used by women because of its soothing effects on the skin, giving your dull, lifeless skin a renewed glow. Parsley essential oil adds a boost of healing properties!

What You Will Need:

½ Cucumber

1 tablespoon Yogurt

2-3 drops Parsley essential oil

What To Do:

1. In a blender, puree the cucumber and yogurt.
2. Add essential oil and mix well.
3. To use, apply to your face evenly. Leave on skin 15 minutes. Rinse off with cool water. Pat dry.

Recipe Variation:

Substitute ½ Avocado for the ½ cucumber in your recipe. Mash avocado until its smooth then apply as directed. You can use fresh parsley if Parsley essential oil is not available.

ROSE PETAL STEAM FACIAL

What You Will Need:

1 handful Rose petals

Water

2 drops Rose essential oil

Pot

What To Do:

1. In a pot, boil the water then remove from heat.
2. Toss in the rose petals. Steep 5 minutes, so that the Rose oil will infuse the water.
3. Stir in the Rose essential oil.
4. Lean over the pot at least 10 inches from the surface and drape towel over your head.
5. Close eyes and steam 5 minutes, taking breaks as needed. Rinse with cool water and pat skin dry.

PEPPERMINT & ROSEMARY STEAM FACIAL

What You Will Need:

4 drops Rosemary essential oil

4 drops Peppermint essential oil

Pot

What To Do:

1. Boil a pot full of water then remove from heat.
2. Stir in the essential oils.
3. Lean over the pot at least 10 inches from the surface with a towel draped over your head.
4. Close eyes and steam 5 minutes, taking breaks as needed. Rinse with cool water and pat skin dry.

SILKY SMOOTH FACIAL WASH

What You Will Need:

1 cup Fresh Cucumber juice

¼ cup Honey

½ cup Plain Yogurt

6 drops Lavender essential oil

4 drops Geranium essential oil

What To Do:

1. In a bowl, mix all of the ingredients.
2. Apply to face just before you bathe. Rinse as normal.

CUSTOM-SCENTED FACIAL MASK

What You Will Need:

1 cup Fine Clay powder

¼ cup Corn Flour

1 tablespoon Ground Oats or another binder

1 tablespoon Dried Skim Milk Powder

1 tablespoon Any Food from "mask ingredients" list

2-5 drops Essential oil (your choice)

Bowl

What To Do:

1. In a bowl, add clay, flour, milk powder and oats.
2. Stir in other mask ingredients and essential oil.
3. Apply clay mixture evenly on the face and neck. Leave on for 10 minutes. Rinse with warm water. Pat skin dry.

Mask & Facial Tips

- To get the most benefits from your mask or facial, make sure your skin is thoroughly clean. You may want to exfoliate or use a facial brush to remove dirt and dead skin cells from the skin's surface. If you prefer, you can also gently steam your face to open pores before applying a mask, so the essential oils will reach down into the skin and go to work.

- Word of Caution: You will most likely see tremendous improvements in your skin after trying a new treatment; however, it may also draw out deep impurities. This will lessen as you continue with your regular regimen.

- Be sure to check if you are allergic to any of the ingredients in your homemade face masks. Do a skin patch test before using it by applying a dab of mask behind your ear. In 5-10 minutes rinse off and check for redness or swelling. If no adverse reaction develops you're good to go!

- Avoid getting your facial mask in your eyes, nose, and mouth.

- Do not use masks that call for salt if you have any open abrasions or scabs.

- Use facial masks only once or twice per week at the most. Follow up with a nourishing moisturizer.

Mask & Facial Tips (continues)

- Standard honey works for facials, but when a recipe calls for it, try to using manuka honey instead.
- Foods that are acidic like lemons, tomatoes and even strawberries will have a more astringent effect. Some fruits may even lighten the skin, so only leave these on for 5 minutes.
- Walnuts and yogurt are both good for using in facial masks when treating acne.
- When using fresh ingredients from home, be sure to use promptly as produce can quickly perish. Do not use your facial treatment if it develops a strange odor or changes color.
- Handle raw eggs with caution. Be sure to wash utensils thoroughly to prevent salmonella contamination.
- Use a shower cap or headband to keep your hair off your face when using your facial mask.
- Only use 1-3 drops of essential oil in your facials or masks.
- There are many good essential oils for facials and masks including: Rosemary, Peppermint, Lemon, Grapefruit, Carrot Seed, Lavender, Geranium, Tea Tree, Chamomile, and Myrtle to name a few.

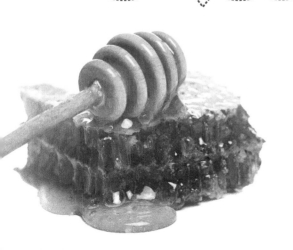

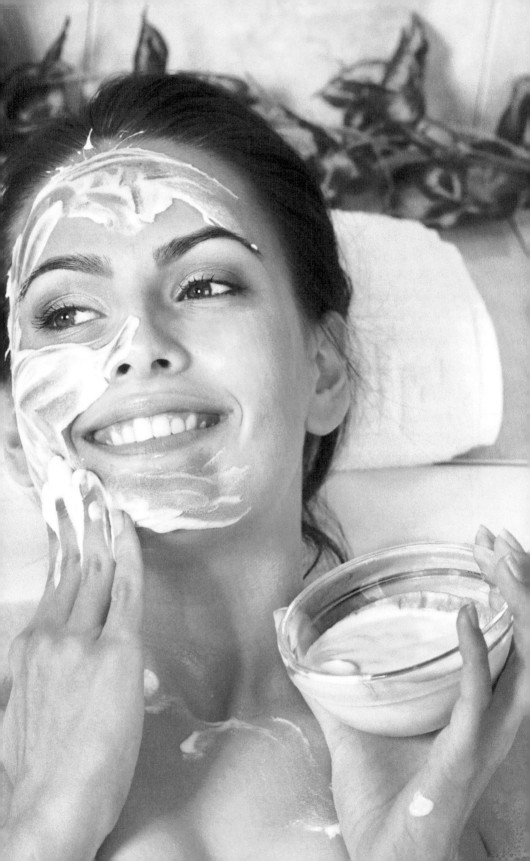

Facial Creams

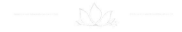

Glossy magazines filled with alluring facial cream ads promise astonishing results like regeneration of skin cells and restored youthfulness—however, not without a hefty price!

Let's face it—overexposure to the sun, dehydration and poor diet really plays havoc on our complexion. The recipes in this section are specifically designed for each skin type and special conditions like acne treatment or wrinkles. Once you have mastered a few of these formulas, feel free to add or delete ingredients that will leave your skin moisturized and nourished with vitamins and minerals.

Now you can achieve those same amazing results for pennies with ordinary ingredients from the kitchen and a few essential oils.

MAYONNAISE FACIAL CREAM

What You Will Need:

2 Fresh Egg Yolks

1 cup Sunflower oil (or substitute Sesame, Safflower oil)

1 tablespoon Wheat Germ oil

1 tablespoon Herb Vinegar

2 drops Rose Geranium essential oil

What To Do:

1. In a bowl, beat the egg yolks. Add the oil very slowly, beating with an electric mixer or blender.
2. As mixture thickens, add vinegar and essential oil. Beat until thick.

3. Apply with upward and outward strokes all over face and throat. Leave on for 20 minutes. Remove with damp cloth and follow with a skin freshener.

ROSE REJUVENATING CREAM

What You Will Need:

1 ounce Beeswax

3 ounces Sweet Almond oil

4 capsules Vitamin E oil (or 10-12 drops)

2 drops Rose essential oil

What To Do:

1. Combine the beeswax, almond oil and vitamin E oil in a pan and heat on low until beeswax is melted.
2. Remove from the heat and whip with a whisk until cool.
3. Add the essential oil and stir to blend well.

SAGGING SKIN NIGHT FORMULA

What You Will Need:

8 drops Geranium essential oil

5 drops Cypress essential oil

5 drops Helichrysum essential oil

1 drop Peppermint essential oil

1 ounce Organic Unscented Lotion

What To Do:

1. In a bottle, add all of the ingredients. Shake well to blend.
2. Apply nightly to the face and neck.

ANTI-WRINKLE CREAM

Mixing and matching essential oils for this recipe creates a natural synergy. Try different essential oils from those listed to find the ones you like best. Since Jojoba oil contains natural wrinkle removing qualities, it works well as the base or carrier oil.

What You Will Need:

2 ounces Jojoba oil or unscented lotion

5 drops Sandalwood essential oil

5 drops Helichrysum essential oil

5 drops Carrot Seed essential oil

5 drops Lavender essential oil

5 drops Frankincense essential oil

Bottle or Jar

What To Do:

1. In a bottle or jar, add 5 drops of each essential oil to the unscented lotion or oil. Stir or shake well to blend.

2. This oil may be used daily or nightly or both for a truly enhancing and youthful appearance.

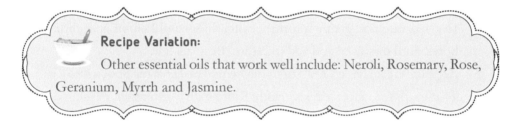

Recipe Variation:

Other essential oils that work well include: Neroli, Rosemary, Rose, Geranium, Myrrh and Jasmine.

ROSEWATER NIGHT CREAM

What You Will Need:

2 ounces Rosewater

1 ounce Glycerin

Bottle

What To Do:

1. In a bottle, mix the Rosewater and glycerin together. Shake well.

2. Apply nightly and work into skin.

LEMON CLEANSING CREAM

This cleansing cream is good for eliminating excess oil and smoothing wrinkles. Plus, the Lemon gives it antiseptic qualities.

What You Will Need:

1 tablespoon Beeswax

3 tablespoons Vegetable oil

1 tablespoon Witch Hazel

1 tablespoon Lemon juice

1/8 teaspoon Borax Powder

6 drops Lemon essential oil

Jar

What To Do:

1. Over low heat, gently melt beeswax in the vegetable oil. Beat for 5 minutes until mixture has a creamy, smooth consistency.
2. In a separate pot, gently warm the witch hazel and Lemon juice. Stir in borax until dissolved and add to cream. Beat steadily.
3. After the cream has cooled, stir in the Lemon essential oil. Spoon into a jar.
4. To use, apply to face with soft cloth. Rinse with warm water. Pat skin dry.

PEPPERMINT CLEANSING CREAM

What You Will Need:

3 tablespoons Olive oil

½ cup Palm oil

4-6 drops Peppermint essential oil

6 drops Onycha essential oil

Bottle

What To Do:

1. In a glass bottle, add all of the ingredients.
2. To use, apply to face with fingers. Remove with tissues. Store in a cool place.

CLEANSING COLD CREAM

This recipe gives you a basic all-purpose cold cream or moisturizer, to which you can add your favorite essential oils, depending on your skin type.

What You Will Need:

52 ounces Beeswax

½ cup Sweet Almond oil

½ teaspoon Borax Powder

¼ cup Rosewater

½-1 teaspoon Essential oils (your choice)

Glass jars

What To Do:

1. Place the beeswax in a double boiler and add the almond oil. Melt the wax over low heat, stirring constantly to combine the ingredients.
2. Remove from heat and dissolve the borax in the rosewater then slowly pour it into the melted wax and oil, whisking constantly. It will turn milky and thicken as it cools.
3. Add essential oils, stirring well.
4. Once it reaches a thick pouring consistency, pour into glass jars or china pots. Makes 7 ounces.

SWEET ORANGE WRINKLE OIL

Use this oil after a day in the sun to replenish your skin's moisture and prevent premature aging.

What You Will Need:

1 teaspoon Sweet Almond oil

2 drops Hazelnut oil

8 drops Orange essential oil

What To Do:

1. In a small bottle, combine all of the ingredients and shake well.
2. To use, cleanse face thoroughly with a cleanser then massage oil into the skin.

ZIT ZAPPER ACNE TREATMENT

What You Will Need:

1 ounce Sweet Almond oil

10 drops Basil essential oil

2 drops Geranium essential oil

3 drops Lavender essential oil

5 drops Tea Tree essential oil

Bottle

What To Do:

1. In a clean bottle, add the carrier oil and essential oils.
2. Close tightly and shake well.
3. To use, apply a small amount to the face, neck or back.

Caution: be certain to avoid the eyes, lips, nostrils and inside the ears.

POND'S CUSTOM-SCENTED COLD CREAM

What You Will Need:

2 tablespoons Carrier oil (such as Hazelnut or Grapeseed oil)

1 tablespoon Beeswax

1 tablespoon Borax Powder

¼ cup Distilled Water

2 capsules Vitamin E oil (or 5-6 drops)

10-12 drops Essential oils (your choice)

Glass jar

What To Do:

1. Place the beeswax in a double boiler and add the carrier oil. Melt the wax over low heat, stirring constantly.
2. Remove from heat. Dissolve the borax in the distilled water. Slowly pour it into the melted wax and oil, whisking constantly. It will turn milky and thicken as it cools.
3. Add the essential oils and Vitamin E oil into the mixture and stir well.

4. Once it reaches a thick pouring consistency, pour into glass jar. Store in a refrigerator until ready for use.

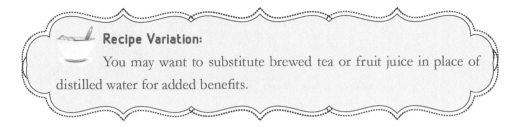

Recipe Variation:

You may want to substitute brewed tea or fruit juice in place of distilled water for added benefits.

CUSTOM-SCENTED COLD CREAM

What You Will Need:

1/3 cup Jojoba oil

2 teaspoons Beeswax

2 tablespoons Cocoa Butter

15-20 drops Essential oils (your choice)

Glass jar

What To Do:

1. Place the beeswax in a double boiler. Stir in the jojoba and cocoa butter. Melt the wax over low heat, stirring constantly.
2. Remove from heat and stir vigorously with a wire whisk until it turns milky and thicken as it cools.
3. Add essential oils into the mixture and blend well.
4. Once it reaches a thick pouring consistency, pour into glass jar. Store in a refrigerator until ready for use.

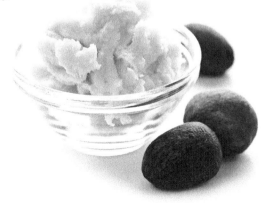

Facial Cream Tips

- Feel free to substitute another carrier oil in any recipe, such as Olive oil or Jojoba oil for the Sweet Almond oil.

- Rosewater can be used in place of distilled water in your recipe to give your facial cream extra moisturizing power. If you prefer a lighter cream, use less Rosewater.

- Store your product in a clean, sterile container with a tight lid to prevent bacteria contamination. After making a product, immediately place it in the refrigerator.

- Be sure to label your container and date it. This will keep you from second-guessing when it was made and its expiration date.

- Don't use your fingers to dig out some of your homemade cream from its container when using it. Instead, use a spoon or another utensil to prevent introducing bacteria from your hands, causing it to spoil faster.

- If you make too much product to use immediately, place the remaining product in a small bottle or container and freeze for later. When you are ready to use it, simply defrost it for a fantastic beauty treat!

- Some of the essential oils you may want to consider for facial creams that fight the effects of aging include: German Chamomile, Carrot Seed, Clary Sage, Fennel, Frankincense, Geranium, Hyssop, Lavender, Myrrh, Neroli, Palmarosa, Rose, Rosemary and Yarrow.

- If you have sensitive skin or a history of allergies, be sure to do a patch test before applying a cream to your face (especially when using new ingredients or essential oils). Simply apply the homemade cream to your forearm in an area about the size of a quarter. Let the cream dry there and cover with a bandage. If there is no reaction within twenty-four hours, it is safe to use.

Facial Toners and Astringents

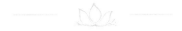

After washing your face with a cleanser, it is important to follow up with a skin toner and/or astringent to ensure complete removal of all soaps. Not only that, the toner will penetrate pores clearing away excess oil, impurities and dead skin cells that the cleanser leaves behind. Toners restore the acid or alkali balance of the skin, refreshing and cooling your skin.

NORMAL TO OILY SKIN TONER

What You Will Need:

½ cup Rosewater

1 drop Juniper Berry essential oil

1 drop Rose Otto essential oil

Dark Glass Bottle

What To Do:

1. Combine all of the ingredients in a clean glass bottle.
2. Shake well before use.

NORMAL TO SENSITIVE SKIN TONER

What You Will Need:

½ cup Chamomile Water

1 drop German Chamomile essential oil

Dark Glass Bottle

What To Do:

1. Combine all of the ingredients in a clean glass bottle.
2. Shake well before use.

NORMAL TO DRY SKIN TONER

What You Will Need:

½ cup Rosewater

1 drop Roman Chamomile essential oil

1 drop Geranium essential oil

Glass Bottle

What To Do:

1. Combine all of the ingredients in a clean glass bottle or container.
2. Shake well before use.

ZESTY MINT SKIN TONER

What You Will Need:

1 cup Witch Hazel

¼ cup White Vinegar

10 drops Peppermint essential oil

10 drops Lemon essential oil

Fresh Mint leaves (optional)

Bottle

What To Do:

1. Add all of the ingredients together in a bottle and shake well.
2. To use, dab on your face with a cotton ball to hydrate skin and remove excess dirt from pores.

LAVENDER APPLE FACIAL TONER

What You Will Need:

1 cup Water

3 drops Lavender essential oil

1 teaspoon Apple Cider vinegar

Spray Bottle

What To Do:

1. Place all of the ingredients in small glass spray bottle. Shake gently.
2. After cleansing the face, spray the toner on cotton pads to use on the face to remove residue the cleanser left behind.

TEA TREE ACNE TONER

This toner is great for spritzing lightly on your face during the day to help remove excess sebum. Carry a small bottle in your handbag so you can use it at work, college, or home.

What You Will Need:

1 cup Water

7 drops Tea Tree essential oil

Spray bottle

What To Do:

1. In a spray bottle, add the water and essential oils together.
2. Shake before each use.

LEMONY LAVENDER TONER

This is a strong acid rinse and is good for oily skin. It tightens pores, soothes sunburn, and can be used as a natural deodorant as well. Mix a fresh batch every 5 days.

What You Will Need:

3 drops Lemon essential oil

3 drops Lavender essential oil

3 teaspoons Distilled Water

¼ cup Lemon juice

Bottle

What To Do:

1. In a small bottle, add all of the ingredients. Shake to mix.

2. Use a soft cotton ball to massage mixture into the skin after cleansing.
3. Rinse immediately with cold water to boost circulation.
4. Use a moisturizer if needed.

AUTUMN BREEZE SKIN TONER

This toner is good for mature skin and helps to reduce wrinkles and slow down the aging process.

What You Will Need:

1 cup Rosewater

3 drops Helichrysum essential oil

3 drops Lavender essential oil

2 drops Frankincense essential oil

2 drops Sandalwood essential oil

1 drop German Chamomile essential oil

Glass bottle

What To Do:

1. In a bottle, add all of the ingredients and shake well.
2. Wait 24 hours to allow the mixture to cure.
3. To use, apply toner using a cotton ball or pad and apply gently to the skin. Don't forget to moisturize afterwards.

SPRING CHICKEN SKIN TONER

This toner is good for normal or combination skin.

What You Will Need:

1 cup Rose Geranium or Lavender Floral Water

5 drops Lavender essential oil

2 drops Rose Geranium essential oil

1 drop Palmarosa essential oil

2 drops Patchouli essential oil

1 drop Ylang Ylang essential oil

Glass bottle

What To Do:

1. In a bottle, add all of the ingredients and shake well.
2. Wait 24 hours to allow the mixture to cure.
3. To use, apply toner using a cotton ball or pad and apply gently to the skin. Don't forget to moisturize afterwards.

ENDLESS SUMMER SKIN TONER

This toner is good for those who have oily skin or are acne prone. It will tighten the pores, remove excess oil and kills the bacteria that causes blackheads.

What You Will Need:

1 cup Witch Hazel

3 drops Palmarosa essential oil

3 drops Tea Tree essential oil

3 drops Petitgrain essential oil

3 drops Lemongrass essential oil

Glass Bottle

What To Do:

1. In a bottle, add all of the ingredients and shake well.
2. Wait 24 hours to allow the mixture to cure.
3. To use, apply toner using a cotton ball or pad and apply gently to the skin. Don't forget to moisturize afterwards.

LAVENDER-GERANIUM TONER

Try this recipe if you have normal to dry skin.

What You Will Need:

2 ounces Green tea

5 drops Lavender essential oil

5 drops Geranium essential oil

Cotton ball or pad

Dark Glass bottle with screw-on lid

What To Do:

1. Make green tea according to package directions.
2. Pour the green tea into a glass bottle, leaving some room at the top.
3. Add five drops of each essential oil to the bottle and shake well.
4. Allow the toner to cool.
5. To use, apply the toner to your freshly-washed face in gentle swipes with a cotton ball or pad. Refrigerate the toner when not using.

CHAMOMILE-SPEARMINT ASTRINGENT

This astringent is especially good for sensitive or very oily skin.

What You Will Need:

½ cup Fresh Mint, chopped or

2 tablespoons Dried Mint

2 tablespoons Dried Chamomile flowers, crushed

10 drops Spearmint essential oil

10 drops German Chamomile essential oil

4 cups Water

Jar

What To Do:

1. Combine all of the ingredients in a small saucepan. Boil for 10 minutes, then remove from heat and allow to steep for 5 minutes.
2. Strain liquid into a jar, cover and refrigerate. It will keep for 2 weeks refrigerated.
3. To use, dab on skin with a cotton ball.

LEMONGRASS ASTRINGENT

This astringent tightens pores, refreshes skin, and removes oils.

What You Will Need:

3 teaspoons Lemon extract

1 Lime, juiced

½ cup Witch Hazel

10 drops Lime essential oil

5 drops Lemongrass essential oil

Jar

What To Do:

1. Combine all of the ingredients in a jar and shake well.

2. Store in the refrigerator for up to 6 months.

SAGE ASTRINGENT

What You Will Need:

4 tablespoons Dried Sage

4 tablespoons Organic Vodka

¼ teaspoon Borax Powder

3 tablespoons Witch Hazel

10 drops Glycerin or Honey

Bottle

What To Do:

1. In a bottle, add the vodka and sage. Steep the sage for 2 weeks then strain.

2. Dissolve borax in witch hazel and stir in the sage/vodka mixture. Add the glycerin.

3. Pour into bottle with a tight cap. Shake before each use.

CUCUMBER-ROSE REFRESHER

This toner will refresh your skin while it tones. It is especially good for sensitive skin and helps as a part of the anti-aging process.

What You Will Need:

3 ounces Fresh Cucumber juice

3 ounces Witch Hazel

1½ ounces Rosewater

What To Do:

1. Mix all of the ingredients together and place in a clean jar. Refrigerate.

2. After cleansing face, soak a clean cotton ball with the toner and gently pat over skin.

TROPICAL FRUIT PUNCH REFRESHER

This citrus blend of Lemon, Lime and Grapefruit is sure to brighten your face!

What You Will Need:

1/2 cup Lemon Yogurt

1 teaspoon Lemon juice

1 teaspoon Lime juice

1 teaspoon Grapefruit juice

2 drops Lemon essential oil

2 drops Lime essential oil

2 drops Grapefruit essential oil

Club Soda

What To Do:

1. Mix all of the ingredients in a bowl.
2. Apply to the face and leave on for 10 minutes.
3. Rinse with cold club soda.

ROSEWATER RINSE

What You Will Need:

1 cup Rose petals

4 drops Rose essential oil

½ cup Witch Hazel

1½ cup Water

What To Do:

1. In a small pan, simmer Rose petals and oil in water for 10 minutes and strain.
2. Add witch hazel to preserve the rinse. Or, refrigerate without preserving. Stores up to 1 week in the refrigerator.

ALOE GEL FOR CONGESTED & INFLAMED SKIN

Soothing Aloe Vera, cleansing Tea Tree and calming Lavender make this a great gel for congested and inflamed skin.

What You Will Need:

1 ounce Aloe Vera gel

1 drop Tea Tree essential oil

1 drop Lavender essential oil

What To Do:

1. In a bowl, mix the Aloe Vera, Tea Tree and Lavender essential oils together.
2. Apply to the skin before applying makeup.

PEPPERMINT SPLASH

This lotion is good for relieving itching!

What You Will Need:

½ cup Water

½ cup Witch Hazel

3-4 drops Peppermint essential oil

Glass Bottle

What To Do:

1. In a bottle, add all of the ingredients. Shake well.
2. Cap and shake well. Apply to skin with a clean cloth.

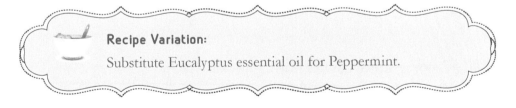

Recipe Variation:
Substitute Eucalyptus essential oil for Peppermint.

HERBAL FACE STEAM

This recipe serves as a deep pore cleanser.

What You Will Need:

1 quart Water

1 handful Herbs

Juice and peel of ½ Lemon

4 drops Lemon essential oil

2 drops Rosemary essential oil

2 drops Lavender essential oil

What To Do:

1. In a pot, bring the water to a boil and add all of the ingredients. Turn off the heat and take the pot to a table.

2. Cover your hair with a shower cap or towel. Drape another towel over your head and the pot, holding your face about 10 inches above the water.

3. Keep your eyes closed and let the steam do its magic cleansing for about 15 minutes. Afterward, rinse with cold water to close the pores.

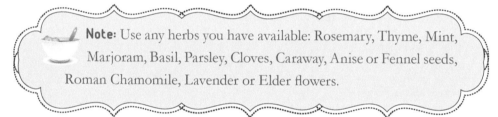

Note: Use any herbs you have available: Rosemary, Thyme, Mint, Marjoram, Basil, Parsley, Cloves, Caraway, Anise or Fennel seeds, Roman Chamomile, Lavender or Elder flowers.

CUSTOM-SCENTED FACIAL TONER

What You Will Need:

1 cup Hydrosol or Floral Water

5-10 drops Essential Oils (your choice)

Bottle

What To Do:

1. Choose essential oils that match your skin type.

2. Choose the hydrosol or floral water you want to use for your blend. For oily/acne prone skin use Witch Hazel; for dry/sensitive skin try Rose water; for normal skin you may want to use Rose Geranium floral water, etc.

3. Add all of the ingredients into a bottle and shake well.

4. Wait 24 hours to allow the mixture to cure.

5. To use, apply toner using a cotton ball or pad and apply gently to the skin. Don't forget to moisturize afterwards.

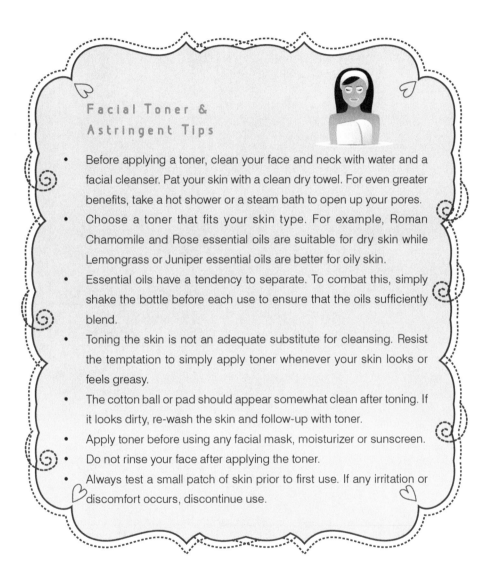

Facial Toner & Astringent Tips

- Before applying a toner, clean your face and neck with water and a facial cleanser. Pat your skin with a clean dry towel. For even greater benefits, take a hot shower or a steam bath to open up your pores.
- Choose a toner that fits your skin type. For example, Roman Chamomile and Rose essential oils are suitable for dry skin while Lemongrass or Juniper essential oils are better for oily skin.
- Essential oils have a tendency to separate. To combat this, simply shake the bottle before each use to ensure that the oils sufficiently blend.
- Toning the skin is not an adequate substitute for cleansing. Resist the temptation to simply apply toner whenever your skin looks or feels greasy.
- The cotton ball or pad should appear somewhat clean after toning. If it looks dirty, re-wash the skin and follow-up with toner.
- Apply toner before using any facial mask, moisturizer or sunscreen.
- Do not rinse your face after applying the toner.
- Always test a small patch of skin prior to first use. If any irritation or discomfort occurs, discontinue use.

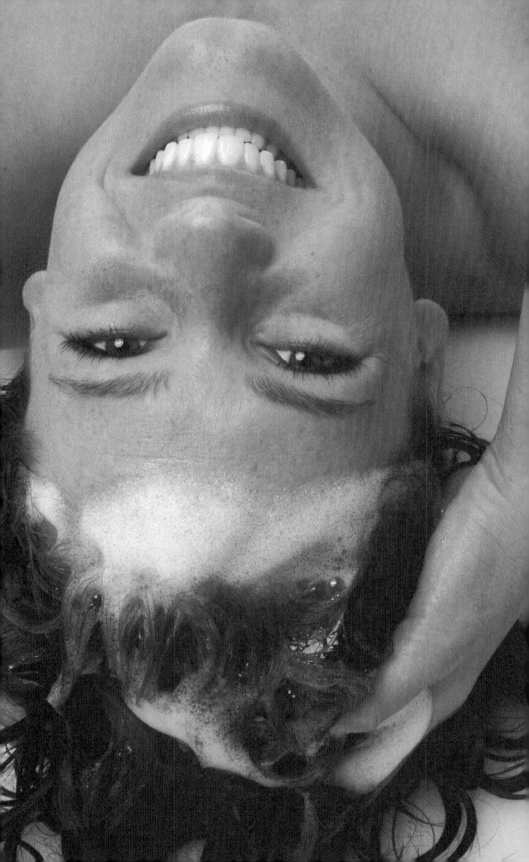

Essential Care for the Hair

Whether you are searching for a method to stimulate more hair growth and/or prevent hair loss, or if you are just looking to make your hair more beautiful and radiant, essential oils added to your hair regimen offer promise.

Discover the most beneficial essential oils for your hair type below to formulate a custom blend of essential oils that will give you that healthy hair you've dreamed about. You can add a little essential oil to your existing hair care product or follow one of the recipes included in this book to create your own signature brand. Either way, you will be reaping the benefits of luxurious hair!

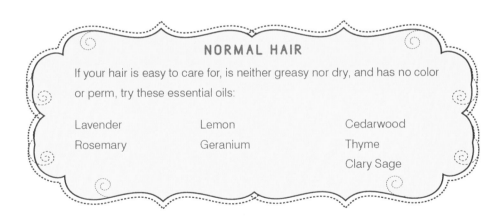

NORMAL HAIR

If your hair is easy to care for, is neither greasy nor dry, and has no color or perm, try these essential oils:

Lavender	Lemon	Cedarwood
Rosemary	Geranium	Thyme
		Clary Sage

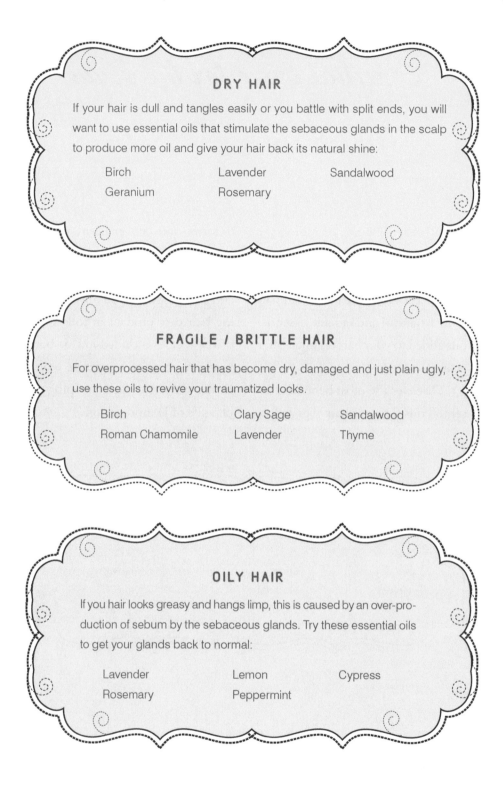

DRY HAIR

If your hair is dull and tangles easily or you battle with split ends, you will want to use essential oils that stimulate the sebaceous glands in the scalp to produce more oil and give your hair back its natural shine:

Birch	Lavender	Sandalwood
Geranium	Rosemary	

FRAGILE / BRITTLE HAIR

For overprocessed hair that has become dry, damaged and just plain ugly, use these oils to revive your traumatized locks.

Birch	Clary Sage	Sandalwood
Roman Chamomile	Lavender	Thyme

OILY HAIR

If you hair looks greasy and hangs limp, this is caused by an over-production of sebum by the sebaceous glands. Try these essential oils to get your glands back to normal:

Lavender	Lemon	Cypress
Rosemary	Peppermint	

SPECIAL HAIR CARE

For treating problems like dandruff, itchy scalp, or even hair loss, essential oils can be very effective. Enrich your hair with the nutrients it needs to minimize hair loss and promote growth.

DANDRUFF

Tea Tree	Birch	Rosemary
Bergamot	Cedarwood	Sage
Patchouli	Cypress	Thyme
Basil	Lavender	Lemon

ITCHY SCALP

Peppermint

STIMULATE GROWTH

Basil	Grapefruit	Rosemary
Cedarwood	Hyssop	Sage
Cypress	Lavender	Thyme
Geranium	Lemon	Ylang Ylang
Ginger		

HAIR LOSS

Birch	Cypress	Sage
Cedarwood	Lavender	Thyme
Roman Chamomile	Lemon	Ylang Ylang
Clary Sage	Rosemary	

Shampoos and Shower Gels

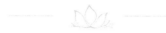

Make every shower delightful with the perfect formula of home-made shampoo or shower gel crafted by you. With only a few botanical extracts and essential oils, you'll be able to avoid all of those fillers and unnecessary chemicals store-bought shampoos contain, leaving your hair and skin super soft and silky smooth. Try a few of these recipes to help replenish and revitalize your hair and skin.

RASPBERRY VANILLA SHOWER GEL

What You Will Need:

½ cup Castile Liquid soap

¼ cup Water

1 teaspoon Salt

7 drops Red Raspberry Seed oil

7 drops Vanilla essential oil

Bottle

What To Do:

1. Combine the liquid soap, water and salt in a bowl and mix.
2. Add essential oils to the mixture and blend well.
3. Store in a container or bottle of your choice.

ROSEMARY CITRUS SHOWER GEL

What You Will Need:

½ cup Castile Liquid soap

½ cup Aloe Vera gel

30 drops Grapefruit essential oil

9 drops Rosemary essential oil

Bottle

What To Do:

1. In a bowl, stir together the liquid soap and Aloe Vera gel.
2. Add essential oils to the mixture. Stir to blend and decant into your bottle of choice.

MARGARITAVILLE SHOWER GEL

What You Will Need:

1 cup Water

1 teaspoon Cornstarch

2 tablespoons Glycerin

1 tablespoon Sweet Almond oil

¼ cup Aloe Vera gel

1 teaspoon Salt

2 capsules Vitamin E oil (or 5-6 drops)

5 drops Lime essential oil

Bottle

What To Do:

1. Place water, cornstarch, glycerin, sweet almond oil, Aloe Vera gel, and salt in a bowl and mix.
2. Add essential oils and the oil from 2 capsules of vitamin E into the mixture and blend well.
3. Pour mixture into a bottle until ready for use.

SENSUAL JASMINE SHOWER GEL

Beautiful moments are born in the shower! This body wash showers you in sensual scents of Jasmine and Vanilla for all-day moisture, giving you smooth skin that's impossible to resist.

What You Will Need:

½ cup Organic Unscented Shampoo

¼ cup Water

¾ teaspoon Salt

7 drops Jasmine essential oil

8 drops Vanilla essential oil

Bottle

What To Do:

1. Pour shampoo, water and salt into a bowl. Stir until it's well mixed.
2. Add the essential oils. Store in a container with lid until use.

ORIENT EXPRESS BATH GEL

What You Will Need:

¼ cup Distilled Water

¼ cup Organic Unscented Shampoo

2 tablespoons Rosewater

1 tablespoon Liquid Glycerin

¾ teaspoon Table Salt

10 drops White Patchouli essential oil

4 drops Mandarin essential oil

Bottle

What To Do:

1. Warm the water and pour into a ceramic bowl.
2. Add the shampoo and stir until well blended.
3. Add the Rosewater, liquid glycerin, salt and essential oils.
4. Stir until well mixed and pour into a bottle.

TANGERINE BODY WASH

What You Will Need:

7 drops Coriander essential oil

10 drops Grapefruit essential oil

7 drops Lavender essential oil

40 drops Tangerine essential oil

4 ounces Organic Unscented Shampoo or Shower gel

Bottle

What To Do:

1. In a bottle, add all of the essential oils and shower gel. You may substitute mild liquid soap or Aloe Vera gel for varying results.
2. Shake well to mix.

FAIRY DUST GLITTER GEL

This fun, whimsical gel is great for your skin. Apply a little after your shower to give your skin sparkle and shine!

What You Will Need:

¼ cup Aloe Vera gel

1 teaspoon Glycerin

¼ teaspoon Fine Glitter

5 drops Lavender essential oil (or your favorite oil)

What To Do:

1. In a small bowl, mix the aloe and glycerin together.
2. Stir in glitter and essential oil. It is ready to use immediately.

FRUIT SMOOTHIE HAIR MASK

This mask is good enough to eat!

What You Will Need:

½ Banana

¼ Avocado

¼ Cantaloupe

1 tablespoon Wheat Germ oil

1 tablespoon Yogurt

2 drops Orange essential oil

What To Do:

1. In a blender, add all of the ingredients and mix.
2. Apply to hair and leave on for 15 minutes. Rinse and wash as normal.

EGG & OLIVE OIL HAIR MASK

Rediscover your hair's natural beauty again with this hair treatment!

What You Will Need:

2 Eggs

4 tablespoons Olive oil

2 drops Rosemary essential oil

Plastic Wrap

What To Do:

1. In a bowl, combine all of the ingredients.
2. Smooth through hair. Wrap hair up with plastic wrap. Leave on hair for 10 minutes. Rinse well.

PEPPERMINT SHAMPOO

This is a tingly treat for all types of hair. It stimulates the scalp without drying.

What You Will Need:

¾ cup Distilled Water

½ cup Organic Unscented Shampoo

1 teaspoon Salt

2 teaspoons Jojoba oil

1/8 teaspoon Peppermint essential oil

1 drop Natural Green Food Coloring (optional)

Bottle

What To Do:

1. Warm the water and pour into a ceramic bowl.

2. Add the shampoo and stir with a wire whisk until well blended.

3. Add the remaining ingredients and stir. Pour into a bottle and close. Makes 8 ½ ounces.

URBAN ALTERNATIVE SHAMPOO

This shampoo is known to be effective in removing impurities such as smog and city grime from the hair.

What You Will Need:

¾ cup Distilled Water

½ cup Organic Unscented Shampoo

1 teaspoon Salt

1 tablespoon Dried Thyme

1 tablespoon Dried Peppermint

1 tablespoon Dried Lavender

1 teaspoon Witch Hazel

1 teaspoon Sweet Almond oil

7 drops Cinnamon essential oil

3 drops Ylang Ylang essential oil

Bottle

What To Do:

1. In a heavy saucepan, bring the water to a boil and add the dried Thyme, Peppermint and Lavender.

2. Remove the pan from the heat and let steep for 30 minutes. Strain the herbs from the water and pour the herbal infused water into a ceramic bowl.

3. Add the shampoo and stir until well mixed. Add the salt, witch hazel, almond oil, Cinnamon and Ylang Ylang essential oils to the mixture, stirring until thick.

4. Bottle and close.

CHAMOMILE FIELDS SHAMPOO

This fresh scent will stay with you all day!

What You Will Need:

4 bags Chamomile tea (or 1 handful Fresh Chamomile flowers)

4 tablespoons Castile soap flakes

4 drops Roman Chamomile essential oil

3 drops Ylang Ylang essential oil

1 ½ tablespoons Glycerin

Bottle

What To Do:

1. Let the tea bags steep in 1 ½ cups of boiling water for 10 minutes.
2. Remove the tea bags. Add the soap flakes and let stand until the soap softens.
3. Stir in glycerin until mixture is well blended.
4. Add the essential oils and blend well. Pour into a bottle.

SOAPWORT SHAMPOO

This recipe will make enough shampoo for 6 washes but needs to be used within 8-10 days.

What You Will Need:

2 cups Water

1 ½ tablespoons Dried Soapwort root, chopped

2 teaspoons Lemon Verbena essential oil

What To Do:

1. Bring the water to a boil. Add Soapwort and simmer, covered for about 20 minutes.
2. Remove from heat and allow to cool. Strain the mixture, keeping the liquid.
3. Add the Lemon Verbena essential oil. Mix well. Pour into a bottle.

CLARIFYING SHAMPOO

Use this amazing shampoo to remove chlorine and other chemicals from your hair and scalp. Rosemary refreshes oily scalps for added volume while the other essential oils stimulate the follicles for new hair growth.

What You Will Need:

2 tablespoons Flax seeds

1 cup Water

2 drops Lemon essential oil

2 drops Rosemary essential oil

2 drops Cedarwood essential oil

2 drops Peppermint essential oil

What To Do:

1. Place flax seeds and water in a saucepan and bring to a boil.
2. Remove from heat and let sit for about 15-20 minutes. Strain and allow the mixture to cool completely.
3. Add the essential oils when cooled. Use once a week for treatment.

HAIR GROWTH / REPAIR SHAMPOO

Get your mane into tiptop shape with this simple recipe. Using warm oil on your scalp eases anxiety and repairs your hair so it looks shiny and glossy! This treatment is also ideal when you want to coax your hair to grow. Plus, Rosemary has been shown to enhance concentration, so if you need to put on your thinking cap, try this treatment for maximum clarity!

What You Will Need:

7 ounces Organic Unscented Shampoo

1 tablespoon Coconut oil

12 drops Clary Sage essential oil

10 drops Ylang Ylang essential oil

12 drops Lavender essential oil

10 drops Rosemary essential oil

Bottle

What To Do:

1. Add the essential oils, coconut oil and unscented shampoo to a bottle.
2. Replace cap and shake well. Shampoo as normal.

ROSEMARY-GERANIUM HAIR CARE SHAMPOO

Now you can have luxury care for dry, damaged hair. This shampoo can be used as a hair mask by leaving on and braiding hair overnight. Rinse in the morning and your hair will be cashmere silk. Be sure to sleep on an old pillowcase!

What You Will Need:

7 ounces Organic Unscented Shampoo

2 tablespoons Coconut oil

15 drops Rosemary essential oil

15 drops Geranium essential oil

15 drops Lavender essential oil

Bottle

What To Do:

1. Add the essential oils, coconut oil, and the unscented shampoo to a bottle.
2. Mix extremely well. Shampoo as normal.

HOT OIL TREATMENT

If you suffer from dry hair, try this aromatherapy recipe to put life back into your parched hair.

What You Will Need:

1 teaspoon Soybean oil

2 teaspoons Castor oil

Few drops Essential oils (your choice)

What To Do:

1. Combine the Soybean and Castor oils and warm on low heat.
2. Add the essential oil of your choice. Stir well.

3. Massage mixture into the scalp and hair. Wrap hair in a hot towel for 15 minutes. Shampoo and rinse out.

CUSTOM-SCENTED SHOWER GEL

Have fun creating your own fragrant shower gel blend! Refer to the section entitled, *Essential Oils for Setting the Mood* for selecting the essential oils best suited for your mood!

What You Will Need:

½ cup Organic Unscented Shampoo

¼ cup Water

¾ teaspoon Salt

15 drops Essential oil (your choice)

Bottle

What To Do:

1. Mix the shampoo and the water in a bowl.
2. Add the salt and essential oil. Stir well. Store in a container with lid.

CUSTOM-SCENTED SHAMPOO

You don't have to be born with great hair. Now you can create a shampoo perfect for yours. Depending on your hair type, choose an essential oil or oils from the chapter, *Essential Care for the Hair* that will give you lustrous hair.

What You Will Need:

¼ cup Distilled Water

¼ cup Castile Soap

½ teaspoon Jojoba oil

6 drops Essential oil (your choice)

Natural Food Coloring (your choice)

Bottle or container

What To Do:

1. Warm the water and pour into a ceramic bowl.
2. Add the soap and jojoba oil, stirring with a wire whisk until well blended.

3. Add the essential oils and natural food coloring (if desired) and stir well.

4. Pour into a bottle and close.

Shampoo & Shower Gel Tips

- Never exceed the suggested amount when adding essential oils to your shampoo and shower gel recipes. Be sure to always know the oils' safety precautions as well—if you don't, then do not use it.

- To enhance the fragrance of your shampoo and shower gels and for eye appeal, add other ingredients such as dried herbs, lavender buds, geranium leaves, rosemary stems, etc. Pulverize them first in a mortar and pestle or food processor. You can also add dried fruit such as orange or grapefruit slices, or spices such as cinnamon sticks, anise star, ground ginger, etc.

- Try using soap scraps melted in water instead of scented store-bought gel or shampoo. A crock pot can be used to melt the soap pieces in water. This takes longer but requires less effort.

- To thicken a runny shampoo mixture add ¼ teaspoon of xanthum gum powder for every cup of shampoo. The powder can be purchased at a local health food store.

- When adding essential oils, remember to wait until the soap cools, as the heat tends to burn off the fragrance somewhat. This will enable you to use less fragrance as well.

- After testing and perfecting your shower gel, make a few extra batches to put in pretty bottles for gift-giving.

- There is a wide range of essential oils scents to choose from. Some of the more popular ones include Vanilla, Coconut, Honeysuckle, Lavender, Rosemary and other herbal scents.

- Add a few drops of Rosemary or Lemongrass essential oils to your store-bought shampoo to boost its conditioning treatment. To keep your hair and scalp healthy, look for hair care products that contain ylang ylang, lavender, rosemary, sandalwood, and geranium essential oils.

- For oily hair, try adding 2-3 drops of Lemon essential oil to a cup of water and use as a final rinse. For dry hair, use Rosemary essential oil instead.

- To reduce dandruff, try making conditioners that contain bergamot, tea tree, or patchouli oil.

- To stimulate hair growth and prevent hair loss, try massaging jojoba, Roman chamomile, or grapefruit oil into the scalp. Leave on for 5 minutes, then rinse.

- To help prevent breakage and get your brush through tangles, sprinkle a few drops of Rosemary essential oil directly on your hairbrush.

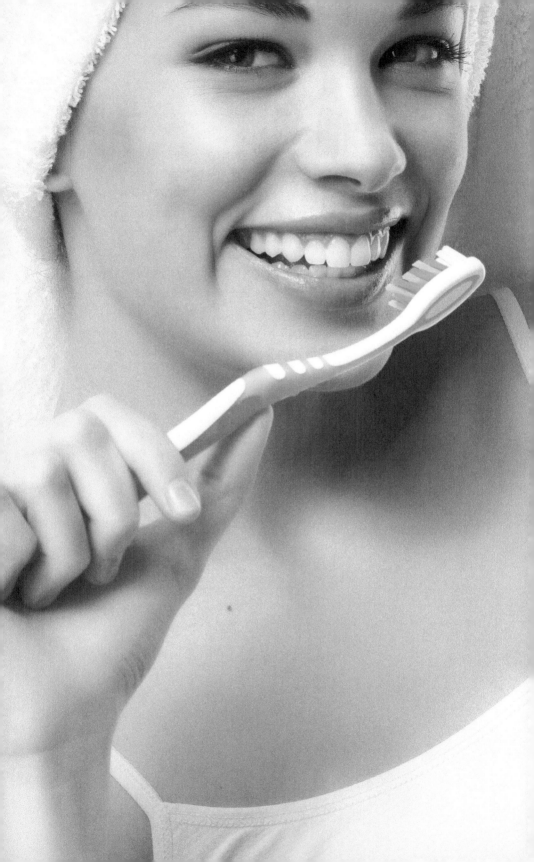

Essential Care for the Mouth

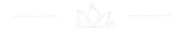

With the growing list of uses for essential oils, it should be no surprise that list includes mouth care. Traditionally, herbs like black walnut, sage and white oak have been used in dental care; today, essential oils serve as a great alternative to commercial products containing fluoride and other harmful chemicals. By making your own natural toothpaste and mouthwash, you can benefit from the essential oil's healing properties: antiseptic, antimicrobial, anti-inflammatory, anti-bacterial, anti-viral, detoxifying and analgesic. Fighting cold sores, canker sores and other unpleasant things including bad breath is a cinch when it comes to nature's own essential oils.

For instance, when you have a toothache or cold sore, don't be afraid to dab a drop of Clove or another safe essential oil straight on. Some of the most commonly used essential oils for dental care include: Peppermint, Clove, Tea Tree, Myrrh, Lemon, Eucalyptus, Rosemary, Spearmint, Wintergreen, Thyme, Oregano, and Helichrysum.

Try these simple recipes that use only a few ingredients and essential oils. Feel free to substitute one or more essential oil, when necessary.

ALL NATURAL TOOTHPASTE

What You Will Need:

¼ teaspoon Peppermint essential oil

¼ teaspoon Spearmint essential oil

¼ cup Arrowroot

¼ cup Orrisroot Powder

¼ cup Water

1 teaspoon Ground Sage

Jar with lid

Spoon

What To Do:

1. Mix all of the dry ingredients in a bowl.

2. Add the essential oils and blend well.

3. Add water until the paste is the desired consistency. Store at room temperature in a tightly covered jar.

4. Dip toothbrush into paste or use a spoon to apply paste to brush. Brush as usual.

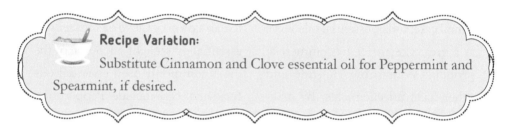

Recipe Variation:

Substitute Cinnamon and Clove essential oil for Peppermint and Spearmint, if desired.

OLD-FASHIONED TOOTH POWDER

What You Will Need:

2 tablespoons Dried Lemon or Orange rind

1 drop Orange essential oil

4 drops Lemon essential oil

¼ cup Baking Soda

1 teaspoon Salt

Small tin or jar with lid

Spoon

What To Do:

1. Place rinds in a food processor and grind until peel becomes a fine powder.

2. Add baking soda and salt, and then process a few seconds more until you have a fine powder.

3. Add essential oils and mix well.

4. Store in an airtight tin or jar.

5. To use, dip moistened toothbrush into mixture or use a spoon to get paste on brush. Brush as usual.

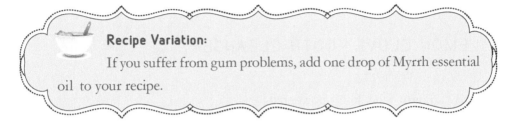

Recipe Variation:

If you suffer from gum problems, add one drop of Myrrh essential oil to your recipe.

SPARKLING TOOTH POWDER

What You Will Need:

4 teaspoons White Clay

1 teaspoon Salt

2 drops Peppermint essential oil

2 drops Lemon essential oil

Small tin or jar

What To Do:

1. Mix all the ingredients until well blended.

2. Store in an airtight jar or tin.

3. To use, dip the toothbrush in the powder mixture, then moisten toothbrush with water and brush as usual.

ULTRA BRIGHT TOOTHPASTE

What You Will Need:

1 teaspoon Baking Soda

¼ teaspoon Hydrogen Peroxide

1 drop Peppermint essential oil

Small tin or container with lid

Spoon

What To Do:

1. Mix all ingredients together to make a paste.

2. Store toothpaste in an airtight jar or container.

3. Dip toothbrush into mixture or use a spoon to get paste onto brush. Brush as usual.

LEMON CLOVE TOOTH CLEANSER

What You Will Need:

Small amount Sage, finely powdered

1 ounce Myrrh, finely powdered

1 pound Arrowroot, powdered

3 ounces Orrisroot powder

20 drops Lemon essential oil

10 drops Clove essential oil

12 drops Bergamot essential oil

Small jar with lid

Spoon

What To Do:

1. In a small bowl, mix all of the dry ingredients together.

2. Add essential oils and blend.

3. Store tooth cleanser in a small jar. Keep closed with lid when not in use.

4. Dip toothbrush into mixture or use a spoon to get paste onto brush and brush as usual.

VANILLA & ROSE GERANIUM TOOTHPASTE

What You Will Need:

½ ounce Chalk, powdered

3 ounces Orrisroot powder

4 teaspoons tincture of Vanilla

15 drops Rose Geranium essential oil

Honey, enough to make a paste

Jar with lid

Popsicle stick or spoon

What To Do:

1. Combine all of the ingredients and mix until you have a smooth paste consistency.

2. Store in an airtight container.

3. Use a clean Popsicle stick or spoon to scoop paste onto brush. Store the stick in same container.

ALCOHOL-FREE ROSEMARY-MINT MOUTHWASH

What You Will Need:

2 ½ cups Distilled or Mineral Water

1 drop Peppermint essential oil

1 drop Rosemary essential oil

1 drop Anise Seed essential oil

Pan

What To Do:

1. Add essential oils to water.

2. Use as a gargle/mouthwash.

3. If you wish to make a larger quantity, double or triple the recipe and add 1 teaspoon of tincture of Myrrh as a natural preservative.

Recipe Variation:

Use Rosemary leaves and Anise seeds if essential oil is not available. Add herbs to boiling water and infuse for 20 minutes. Peppermint leaves can be substituted for essential oil as well.

SPEARMINT-ALOE MOUTHWASH

What You Will Need:

6 ounces Water

2 ounces Organic Vodka

4 teaspoons Liquid Glycerin

1 teaspoon Aloe Vera gel

10-15 drops Spearmint essential oil

Bottle

What To Do:

1. Boil the water and vodka.
2. Add glycerin and Aloe Vera gel. Remove from the heat and let cool slightly.
3. Add Spearmint essential oil and stir well.
4. Pour into bottle, cap tightly. Use as usual.

ALCOHOL-FREE ANISE MOUTHWASH

What You Will Need:

1 cup Distilled Water

2 drops Peppermint essential oil

2 drops Spearmint essential oil

1 drop Anise essential oil

1 teaspoon Honey

1 teaspoon Fresh Lemon juice

Glass Bottle

What To Do:

1. In a small bowl, add honey, lemon juice and essential oils. Stir to mix well.
2. Add water to the honey mixture, until the honey is dissolved.
3. Pour the mixture into a bottle and shake well before use.

PEPPERMINT & THYME MOUTHWASH

What You Will Need:

6 tablespoons Organic Vodka

10 drops Peppermint or Fennel essential oil

2 drops Lemon juice

1 drop Thyme or Chamomile essential oil

Glass Bottle

What To Do:

1. Pour the alcohol into a clean sterilized glass bottle or jar.
2. Add the essential oils one at a time and shake well.
3. To use, add a few teaspoons to a glass of warm water and swish around in mouth. Store in the refrigerator for a longer shelf-life.

CINN-A-MINT MOUTHWASH

This mouthwash soothes and invigorates the gums. Great for canker sores too.

What You Will Need:

1 cup Water

1 teaspoon Organic Vodka

2 drops Cinnamon essential oil

2 drops Spearmint essential oil

1 drop Peppermint essential oil

2 drops Tea Tree essential oil

Glass Bottle

What To Do:

1. Pour the alcohol into a clean sterilized glass bottle or jar.
2. Add the essential oils one at a time and shake well.
3. To use, add a few teaspoons to a glass of warm water and swish around in mouth. Store in the refrigerator for a longer shelf-life.

ANTI-PLAQUE MOUTHWASH

This mouthwash contains the essential oils of Tea Tree, Myrrh, Clove and Cardamom, which are all germicidal. Myrrh is also anti-inflammatory, while Cardamom prevents plaque from sticking to the teeth.

What You Will Need:

16 drops Tea Tree essential oil

2 drops Myrrh essential oil

1 drop Clove essential oil

1 drop Cardamom essential oil

Bottle

What To Do:

1. In a small bottle, add all of the essential oils. Replace top and shake well to blend.

2. Place 2 drops on your toothbrush with toothpaste and brush as usual. Or, place 2 drops in a shot glass full of water and use as a mouthwash (try not to swallow, but it won't hurt you if you do).

CUSTOM-SCENTED MOUTHWASH

This homemade mouthwash recipe is not only inexpensive without the harsh chemicals, but it is also alcohol-free.

What You Will Need:

1 teaspoon Salt

1 teaspoon Baking Soda

8 ounces Water

1-2 drops Essential oils (your choice)

Bottle

What To Do:

1. In a pan, boil water then remove from heat.

2. Add baking soda, salt and essential oils. Stir well.

3. Pour mixture into a sterilized bottle. Use as normal.

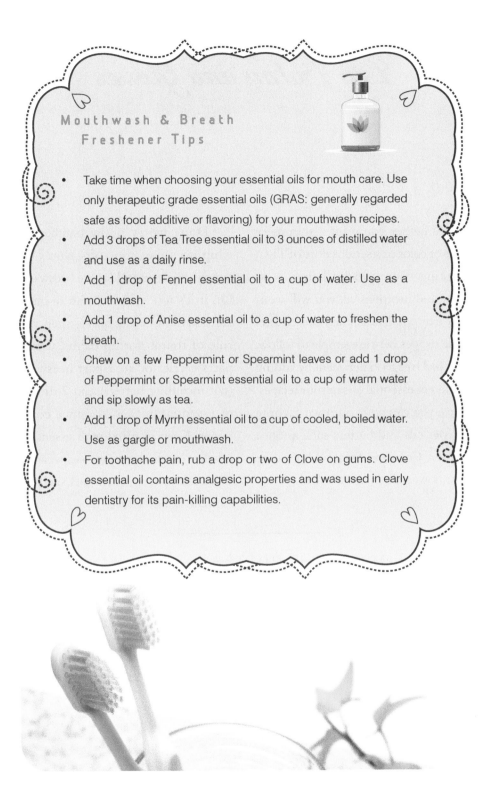

Mouthwash & Breath Freshener Tips

- Take time when choosing your essential oils for mouth care. Use only therapeutic grade essential oils (GRAS: generally regarded safe as food additive or flavoring) for your mouthwash recipes.
- Add 3 drops of Tea Tree essential oil to 3 ounces of distilled water and use as a daily rinse.
- Add 1 drop of Fennel essential oil to a cup of water. Use as a mouthwash.
- Add 1 drop of Anise essential oil to a cup of water to freshen the breath.
- Chew on a few Peppermint or Spearmint leaves or add 1 drop of Peppermint or Spearmint essential oil to a cup of warm water and sip slowly as tea.
- Add 1 drop of Myrrh essential oil to a cup of cooled, boiled water. Use as gargle or mouthwash.
- For toothache pain, rub a drop or two of Clove on gums. Clove essential oil contains analgesic properties and was used in early dentistry for its pain-killing capabilities.

Lip Balms and Glosses

Whether you want a shimmery kiss of color or a serious dose of TLC, making your own lip balms is so easy and inexpensive, you will wonder why you hadn't tried this before! The recipes here are simple to follow, but feel free to experiment by adding different essential oils in your recipes. Plus, you can add your own favorite carrier oils and butters such as Shea butter, Coconut, Sweet Almond or Sunflower oil to name a few!

Don't worry if the batch you whip up seems too soft—you can simply reheat and add more beeswax. Or, if it's too hard, you can re-melt and add more carrier oil. As a general rule of thumb for lip balms, use 3 parts carrier oil to 1 part beeswax (not including butters) and 2 drops of essential oil per ¼-ounce container. Keep in mind with essential oils less is always more—especially when it comes to warm oils such as Cinnamon and Clove!

ORANGE-MANGO LIP BUTTER

Make your own lip balm for a softer, smoother finish. This one will instantly hydrate your lips.

What You Will Need:

4 teaspoons Olive oil

1 teaspoon Beeswax, grated

2 teaspoons Mango butter

15 drops Orange essential oil

1 capsule Vitamin E oil (or 2-3 drops)

Containers

What To Do:

1. Melt the beeswax, mango butter, and olive oil in a double boiler.
2. Allow to cool slightly then add essential oil and Vitamin E oil. Stir well.
3. Pour into clean containers.

ZESTY LIME LIP BALM

This recipe makes 8-9 lip balm tubes or tins!

What You Will Need:

2 tablespoons Sunflower oil

1 tablespoon and 1 teaspoon Beeswax

1 tablespoon Coconut oil

10 drops Lime essential oil

Tins or lip tubes

What To Do:

1. Pour the sunflower and coconut oil into a glass measuring cup. Add beeswax and melt in a microwave or double boiler.
2. When melted, add essential oil and stir with a popsicle stick.
3. While still hot, pour the mixture into small tins or lip balm tubes.

MINT-CHOCOLATE LIP BALM

What You Will Need:

1 tablespoon Beeswax

1/8 cup Coconut oil

½ tablespoon Shea butter

½ tablespoon Cocoa butter

½ teaspoon Honey

1 teaspoon Cocoa powder

2 capsules Vitamin E oil (or 5-6 drops)

3 drops Peppermint essential oil

What To Do:

1. Place the Shea butter, cocoa butter and coconut oil in a small pot or double boiler. Heat over very low heat for 20 minutes, stirring occasionally.

2. Add the beeswax and stir well.

3. After the beeswax has completely melted, remove from heat and add the essential oil, honey, vitamin E, and cocoa powder, whisking well the whole time.

4. After everything is incorporated and smooth, transfer to a lip balm tube or tin and allow to set for 3 hours.

HEMP OIL LIP BALM

What You Will Need:

3 tablespoons Coconut oil

1 tablespoon Castor oil

1 tablespoon Sunflower oil

1 tablespoon Hemp Seed oil

1 tablespoon Beeswax

1 tablespoon Honey

10-12 drops Spearmint essential oil

Tins or containers

What To Do:

1. Melt the beeswax and coconut oil together in a microwave or in a double boiler.

2. Add honey and heat slightly, stirring constantly.

3. Add the sunflower and caster oils.

4. As the mixture begins to thicken add the Hemp Seed oil and essential oil. Stir constantly until it thickens.

5. Pour balm mixture into small containers and let cool.

SWEET ALMOND LIP GLOSS

Try this pampering balm for a smooth finishing touch!

What You Will Need:

2 teaspoons Beeswax

3-6 drops Vanilla essential oil

3-6 drops Neroli essential oil

1 teaspoon Sweet Almond oil

3 drops Honey

1½ teaspoon Cocoa butter

1 capsule Vitamin E oil (or 2-3 drops)

What To Do:

1. In a glass measuring cup, add beeswax, sweet almond oil, honey, cocoa butter and vitamin E oil.
2. Heat on high in a microwave at 30-second increments or in a double boiler until melted. Mix well.
3. Remove from heat and add essential oils, stirring thoroughly.
4. Immediately pour into small tins or lip balm tubes.

COLD SORE RELIEF BALM

This one is good for healing cold sores or fever blisters.

What You Will Need:

1 ounce Emu oil

1 ounce Sweet Almond oil

1 ounce Avocado oil

½ ounce Beeswax

¼ ounce Aloe Vera gel

6 drops Lavender essential oil

2 drops Tea Tree essential oil

3 drops Lime essential oil

Tin or small container

What To Do:

1. Combine Emu, sweet almond, avocado, Aloe Vera, and beeswax in a glass measuring cup.
2. Heat in the microwave on high in 30-second increments until melted or in a double boiler on the stovetop. Stir well.
3. Remove from heat and add essential oils. Blend thoroughly.
4. Pour mixture into small tins or lip balm tubes. Let harden.
5. To use, apply at the first sign of a cold sore or blister.

GRAPEFRUIT LIP BALM

What You Will Need:

1 tablespoon Cocoa butter

2 tablespoons Sweet Almond oil

1 tablespoon Olive oil

1 tablespoon & 1 teaspoon Beeswax

5-10 drops Grapefruit essential oil

Tins or containers

What To Do:

1. In a small microwave-safe glass dish, add the Cocoa butter, sweet almond, olive oil, and beeswax. Microwave on high in 30-second increments until mixture becomes a liquid.
2. When melted and slightly cooled, add the Grapefruit essential oil.
3. Pour into lip pots to harden.

RED HOT LIP SCRUB

During the winter months, this lip scrub is great for exfoliating your chapped, dry, sore lips. Pucker up!

What You Will Need:

½ tablespoon Raw Sugar

1 ½ tablespoon Brown Sugar

1 drop Vanilla essential oil

8-10 drops Cinnamon essential oil

Tin or small container

What To Do:

1. In a bowl, mix all of the ingredients together.
2. Store in a small container.
3. To use, dig some out with your finger and scrub mixture on lips in a circular motion. Rinse off.

LEMON COCONUT LIP BALM

This recipe will fill 8-9 lip balm tubes!

What You Will Need:

1 tablespoon Coconut oil

2 tablespoons Sunflower oil

1 tablespoon & 1 teaspoon Beeswax

10 drops Lemon essential oil

9 Lip balm tubes or containers

What To Do:

1. Melt the beeswax in a glass measuring cup in the microwave or in a double boiler over low heat until melted.
2. Add coconut and sunflower oils. Stir well.
3. Remove from heat and stir in essential oil.
4. Let balm cool slightly and pour into containers. For a softer lip balm, add more oil. For a harder lip balm, add more beeswax.

COOL MINT LIP BALM

What You Will Need:

1 tablespoon Cocoa Butter

2 tablespoons Sweet Almond oil

1 tablespoon Olive oil

1 tablespoon & 1 teaspoon Beeswax

5-10 drops Peppermint essential oil

Tins or lip balm tubes

What To Do:

1. Melt the cocoa butter and beeswax slowly in a double boiler on the stove, until melted.

2. Add carrier oils and stir well.

3. Add Peppermint essential oil, a few drops at a time, for taste. Gently reheat if needed.

4. Cool slightly before pouring into containers. To test consistency, place a drop on a spoon and set in the refrigerator to cool for a few minutes. Test on your lips. For a softer lip balm, add more oil. For a harder lip balm, add more beeswax.

CREAMY VANILLA LIP BUTTER

This creamy lip balm recipe is a lot of fun to make! You can make just one kind, or you can experiment and create several different flavors. Lip balm makes a great addition to gift baskets!

What You Will Need:

1 tablespoon Beeswax

½ tablespoon Cocoa butter

4 teaspoons Sweet Almond oil

1 teaspoon Honey (optional)

1 capsule Vitamin E oil (or 2-3 drops)

5-10 drops Vanilla essential oil

What To Do:

1. Place the beeswax, cocoa butter, and sweet almond oil in a heat-proof measuring cup. For a sweeter lip gloss, add 1 teaspoon of honey.

2. Place the measuring cup in 1 inch of hot water in a large frying pan on low heat.

3. Stir the mixture in the measuring cup with a popsicle stick or bamboo skewer every couple of minutes until the wax is completely melted (about 15-20 minutes). Remove from heat.

4. Stir in vitamin E oil and essential oil.

5. Pour the mixture into lip balm dispensers, containers, or small jars. This recipe will fill 4-5 containers. You may find it easier (and cleaner) to either use a small dropper to transfer the mixture into the small containers, or to use a small funnel to pour the mixture.

> **Extra Ideas:**
> To make this lip balm into a softer, shinier lip gloss, try adding a teaspoon more sweet almond oil, and a teaspoon less beeswax (or experiment with your own proportions to find something you like). Create fun labels for your lip balm creations!

LUSCIOUS LAVENDER LIP BALM

What You Will Need:

4 tablespoons Jojoba, Sweet Almond, or Olive oil

1 tablespoon Beeswax

1 teaspoon Honey

3 capsules Vitamin E oil (or 8-9 drops)

7 drops Lavender essential oil (or another essential oil)

1 teaspoon Cocoa Powder

1-2 drops Natural Red Food Coloring

What To Do:

1. Warm the oils, beeswax and honey in a small, stainless steel pot or bowl. Be sure to warm it on very low heat. You can also use a double boiler.

2. Stir until the beeswax is completely melted.

3. Remove from heat and quickly whisk in the essential oil, vitamin E, cocoa powder, and natural food coloring.

4. Place the bottom of the bowl into a shallow pan of ice water and continue whisking quickly as you add the honey. Once the honey is incorporated,

quickly transfer the balm into your lip balm container and allow to set for 3 hours.

PINK PETAL LIP BALM

This not-quite red balm pampers your lips with a lightweight splash of color!

What You Will Need:

2 tablespoons Coconut oil

1 tablespoon Cocoa butter

1 tablespoon Dried Rosebuds (or dried flowers, green tea, etc.)

3 capsules Vitamin E oil (or 8-9 drops)

3 drops Rose essential oil (or substitute Lavender, Vanilla, or Orange)

3 drops Natural Red Food Coloring

What To Do:

1. In a stainless steel bowl or pot, melt the coconut oil on low heat.
2. After the oil has liquefied, add your roses (or other dried flowers) and stir well. Allow to steep on very low heat for 1 hour.
3. Strain oil into a bowl through a fine-mesh sieve or cheesecloth. Wipe out your original heating pot/bowl, pour oil back in, and return to heat.
4. Add cocoa butter and stir until melted. Remove from heat. Add vitamin E oil, essential oil and natural food coloring. Stir well.
5. Transfer to a small container and let set for 3 hours or until completely set.

APRICOT-ORANGE LIP BALM

Get smoother, softer looking lips with this balm!

What You Will Need:

1 teaspoon Beeswax

1 teaspoon Apricot Kernel oil

1 teaspoon Calendula oil

3-5 drops Orange essential oil

Small container

What To Do:

1. Using a double boiler, melt the beeswax.

2. Add the apricot and calendula oils, stirring constantly.

3. Remove from the heat while stirring and when partly cooled, add the essential oils.

4. Store in a small container.

CUSTOM LIP BALM

This large recipe makes enough to fill 24 ¼-ounce lip balm containers!

What You Will Need:

1 ounce Sweet Almond or Apricot Kernel oil

1 ounce Sunflower oil

1 ounce Avocado or Olive oil

1 ounce Shea butter

¼ ounce Beeswax

30-40 drops essential oils (your choice)

6-8 drops Natural Red Food Coloring

What To Do:

1. Melt the beeswax, Shea butter and oils using a double boiler or a pan on very low heat. When beeswax is completely melted, remove from heat and allow to cool.

2. Add 30-40 drops of essential oil and natural food coloring, if desired.

3. Increase the amount of beeswax to ½ ounce if you like your lip balm more solid.

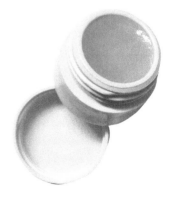

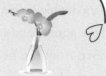

Lip Balm & Gloss Tips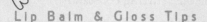

- Choose essential oils that are GRAS (generally regarded as safe as a food additive).
- Try different oils on your lips to choose the best one for your skin and taste preference.
- If the balm is too hard (waxy), add more oil to your mixture. If it is too soft, add more wax.
- Add a few drops of homemade food coloring (for instance, made with beet juice or another fruit) for a natural matte red color. Or, shave off a little from an old lipstick for that cinematic color. Only use natural food coloring, as it may be alcohol-based.
- For healing balms, try essential oils like Comfrey, Rosemary, Tea Tree or Camphor, which have excellent healing properties.
- Discard old lip gloss if it changes color, odor, or texture.
- Use candy melts to color the gloss and make it taste sweet.
- If you're not into scrubs for the lips, the editors of beauty magazines suggest a baby toothbrush for smoothing out lips.
- Recycle old lip gloss or balm containers. Other places to look for interesting containers include craft stores, bead shops, or fishing tackle supplies.

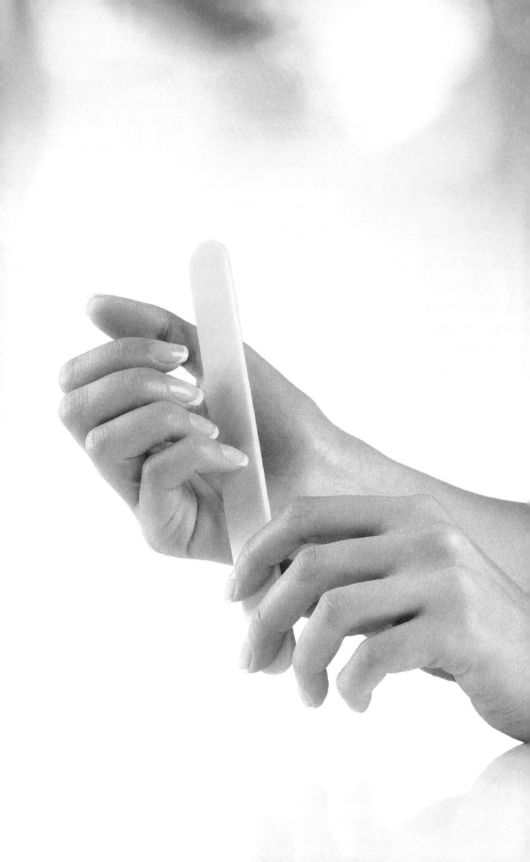

Essential Care for the Hands and Nails

Presenting your perfect ten—your hands and nails—is very important. A good manicure is a basic ingredient in the package of looking your best. No matter whether your nails are long and polished with a hip new color or simply shaped and buffed, well-cared-for hands will feel great and give you that boost of confidence.

Believe it or not, one of the first things people look at when they meet you, besides your face, are your hands. Even when you're wearing your hair in the latest style or look fabulous in those to-die-for jeans, top celebrity nail-care experts agree—if your nails are not done, you're not done! And the truth is, it is probably the one place on your body you will see most often.

Your nails will greatly benefit from essential oils' nourishing and healing properties, enhancing their appearance. The nail butter and oil treatment recipes found in this section will not only strengthen your nails preventing them from becoming brittle, but will also cure common nail problems like fungus. Try one of these recipes as part of nail care regimen or mix together your own formula to keep your nails in tiptop shape.

WEAK NAIL STRENGTHENING OIL

This recipe is great for strengthening weak, thin nails!

What You Will Need:

10 drops Frankincense essential oil

10 drops Lemon essential oil

10 drops Myrrh essential oil

2 tablespoons Wheat Germ oil

Small dark glass bottle

What To Do:

1. Combine all of the ingredients in a small, dark glass bottle.
2. Apply with cotton swab or paint brush to bare nails twice a day.

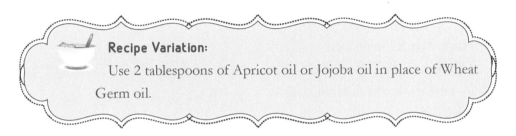

Recipe Variation:

Use 2 tablespoons of Apricot oil or Jojoba oil in place of Wheat Germ oil.

WHITENING NAIL SCRUB

What You Will Need:

1 tablespoon Lemon juice

1 drop Lemon essential oil

Baking Soda

Small bowl

What To Do:

1. In a small bowl, add juice, essential oil and baking soda to form a paste.
2. Massage into nails, then rinse well.

SWEET 'N SOUR NAIL GROWTH OIL

What You Will Need:

20 drops Lavender essential oil

10 drops Lemon essential oil

2 tablespoons Sweet Almond oil

Small dark glass bottle

What To Do:

1. In a bottle, add the almond oil and the essential oils.
2. Tighten the cap and shake the bottle vigorously for one minute to blend.
3. To use, massage the nail bed once a day to encourage healthy growth.

STIMULATING NAIL GROWTH RUB

What You Will Need:

1 drop Peppermint essential oil

1 drop Myrrh essential oil

2 drops Lavender essential oil

1½ tablespoon Sweet Almond oil

Small dark glass bottle

What To Do:

1. In a bottle, add the almond oil and the essential oils.
2. Shake the bottle vigorously for 1 minute to blend.
3. Rub into cuticles and onto nails once a day at bedtime.

ROSE CUTICLE OIL

What You Will Need:

¼ cup Sweet Almond carrier oil

2 teaspoons Apricot Kernel oil

5 drops Geranium essential oil

2 drops Rose essential oil

Small dark glass bottle

What To Do:

1. Mix all of the ingredients together and store in a dark colored bottle.
2. To use, massage into nails every day. Add a few drops to a dish of warm water and soak for 10 minutes to encourage healthy growth.

LEMON CITRUS SOAK

Lemons have been used for hand and nail care for centuries. Lemon juice and the essential oil of Lemon whitens nails while stimulating healthy growth. Try this refreshing citrus soak.

What You Will Need:

8 ounces Spring water

1 tablespoon Aloe Vera gel

10 drops Lemon essential oil

What To Do:

1. Mix all of the ingredients in a small bowl.
2. Soak fingertips for 10 minutes.
3. Wash hands as normal.

SIMPLE OLIVE CUTICLE OIL

Cuticle oils made at home are easy and beneficial to your nails. Keeping cuticles hydrated and healthy lead to harder, faster growing, well-maintained nails. Be sure to add some essential oils in the blend for the extra nourishment.

What You Will Need:

2 tablespoons Olive oil

10 drops Essential Oils (your choice)

What To Do:

1. In a small bowl, combine both ingredients. Mix well.
2. To use, apply a very small amount to each cuticle and work into the cuticle, nail and surrounding skin. Olive oil absorbs nicely into the skin after a few minutes and is great for elbows as well.

TEA TREE CUTICLE OIL

What You Will Need:

10 drops Tea Tree essential oil

2 tablespoons Sweet Almond oil

Small dark glass bottle

What To Do:

1. Combine oils in a small bottle and replace cap. Shake to blend.
2. Warm up oil before use by running bottle under warm water.
3. Apply over entire nail bed and surrounding skin and cuticles.

ANTI-AGING CUTICLE OIL

What You Will Need:

10 drops Carrot Seed essential oil

2 tablespoons Jojoba oil

Small dark glass bottle

What To Do:

1. Combine oils in a small bottle and replace cap. Shake to blend.
2. Warm up oil by running bottle under warm water.
3. Apply over entire nail bed and surrounding skin and cuticles.

HEALING CUTICLE OIL

Hemp Seed oil is said to aid in the healing of skin lesions, dry skin, and inflammation of the skin and joints.

What You Will Need:

5-10 drops Tea Tree essential oil

2 tablespoons Hemp Seed oil

Small dark glass bottle

What To Do:

1. Combine oils in a small bottle. Shake to blend.
2. Warm up oil by running bottle under warm water.
3. Apply over entire nail bed and surrounding skin and cuticles. There is no need to wash off.

NAIL BUTTER

What You Will Need:

2 tablespoons Beeswax

2 tablespoons Cocoa Butter

3 tablespoons Jojoba oil

1 tablespoon Grapeseed oil

4 drops Rose essential oil

4 drops Carrot Seed essential oil

4 drops Rosemary essential oil

4 drops Geranium essential oil

4 drops Sandalwood essential oil

What To Do:

1. Combine the beeswax, cocoa butter and carrier oils in saucepan and warm on low heat until cocoa butter and beeswax have melted.
2. Remove from heat. Add the essential oils, stirring well.
3. Let cool slightly and pour into jars.
4. To apply, use a cotton swab or orange stick to get a small amount of the cream out. Apply to the nails and massage with your fingers.

LADY'S MANTLE HAND LOTION

What You Will Need:

2 tablespoons Lady's mantle (strong infusion)

2 tablespoons Glycerin

2 teaspoons Irish moss, melted in a little hot water

4 tablespoons Organic Vodka

10 drops Rose or Geranium essential oil

Small dark glass bottle

Bowl

What To Do:

1. In a bowl, add glycerin into melted moss.
2. Add essential oils to the vodka, and blend into the glycerin mixture.

3. Stir in Lady's mantle infusion and mix well.

4. Pour into a jar and cap tightly. Shake before using.

HONEY-ROSEWATER HAND LOTION

What You Will Need:

1 tablespoon Irish moss

¼ cup Rosewater

¼ cup Honey

½ cup Water

1/3 cup Glycerin

1 drop Rose essential oil

Jar or container with lid

What To Do:

1. In a pan, combine the water and Irish moss, and simmer over low heat until the mixture is thick—about 10 minutes.

2. Strain the mixture to remove the Irish moss.

3. Combine the strained liquid with the remaining ingredients. Makes about 1 cup.

HEAVY DUTY GARDENERS' HAND CREAM

What You Will Need:

2 tablespoons Beeswax

½ teaspoon Carnuba wax

2 tablespoons Jojoba oil

1 teaspoon Aloe Vera gel

4 capsules Vitamin E oil (or 10-12 drops)

1 drop Lavender essential oil

Jar or container with lid

What To Do:

1. Melt the first 4 ingredients in a stainless steel pot on the stove or use a glass measuring cup in the microwave.

2. Remove from heat and beat until cool, adding the vitamin E oil before mixture thickens. Continue beating until the mixture becomes creamy.

3. Add a drop of Lavender or another favorite essential oil and continue beating until cream has completely cooled.

4. Spoon your cream into a jar and store in a cool dark place.

SUMMER FIELDS HAND CREAM

What You Will Need:

1 cup Aloe Vera gel

1 teaspoon Lanolin

1 teaspoon Vitamin E oil

1/3 cup Coconut oil

½-¾ ounce Beeswax

¾ cup Sweet Almond oil

½ teaspoon Lavender essential oil

½ teaspoon Rose Geranium essential oil

Glass Jars

What To Do:

1. Place the Aloe Vera gel, lanolin, and vitamin E oil in blender or food processor to blend.

2. Place the coconut oil and beeswax in 2-cup glass measuring cup and microwave on high 30 seconds. Stir and continue heating in 10-second increments until fully melted.

3. Stir in the sweet almond oil, reheating if necessary. Run blender or processor at low to medium speed and pour in melted oils in a thin stream.

4. As oil is blended in, the cream will turn white and blender's motor will start to grind. As soon as the melted oils are added and you've achieved mayonnaise-like consistency, stop motor, add essential oils and pulse-blend. Do not over blend.

5. Transfer cream to glass jars while still warm, because it thickens quickly.

HONEY-ALMOND CLEANSING CREAM

This cream has a slightly oily texture and can be used for applying as a conditioner to the hands before doing outside work, such as gardening.

What You Will Need:

¼ cup Honey

¼ cup Vegetable shortening

1 tablespoon Almonds, grounded

1 teaspoon Liquid Lecithin

2 tablespoons Bee Pollen

1 Egg Yolk, room temperature

1 teaspoon Rosewater

2 drops Orange essential oil

Jar or container with lid

What To Do:

1. In a jar, combine all of the ingredients and mix well.
2. Use as a cold cream for dry skin or for sunburn. Makes about ¾ cup.

SOY WAX HAND TREATMENT

What You Will Need:

4 ounces Soy Wax

1 ounce Sweet Almond oil

20 drops Lavender essential oil

Olive oil

Double boiler

Sandwich bags

What To Do:

1. Melt the Soy wax, almond oil, and essential oil in a double boiler. Be sure to use a double boiler for safety purposes.
2. Carefully pour the wax into a dish and wait until a skin has formed on the top of the wax. When this happens, the temperature should be about right for submerging your hands. But before you do, be sure to test the

wax for comfort in case it is still a little too warm. Testing a little on your wrist usually works.

3. Wash your hands and pat dry with paper towel.

4. Smooth on the olive oil and be sure to cover every inch of your hands and fingers. Dip each hand into the wax repeatedly until you have several layers of wax built up on your hands.

5. Have someone help you put the sandwich bags on each hand and wait for about 30 minutes.

6. To remove wax, simply peel it away starting at the wrist and pulling down. It should come off in large sections. Gently massage both hands and you are done.

CUSTOM-SCENTED NAIL & CUTICLE OIL

What You Will Need:

10 drops Essential oil (your choice)

2 tablespoons Carrier oil (your choice)

Small dark glass bottle

What To Do:

1. Combine oils in a small bottle and replace cap. Shake to blend.

2. Warm up oil by running bottle under warm water.

3. Apply over entire nail bed and surrounding skin and cuticles.

CUSTOM-SCENTED HAND CREAM

What You Will Need:

¼ cup Beeswax

½ cup Sweet Almond oil

½ cup Coconut oil

¼ cup Rosewater (or another floral water)

Essential oils (your choice)

Jar or container with lid

What To Do:

1. Melt the beeswax and coconut oil in a double boiler (or microwave).

2. Add the remaining ingredients and heat for several minutes until well mixed.

3. Pour into a container while still hot since it thickens as it cools. Makes about 1 ½ cups.

4. Store in a jar or container until ready for use.

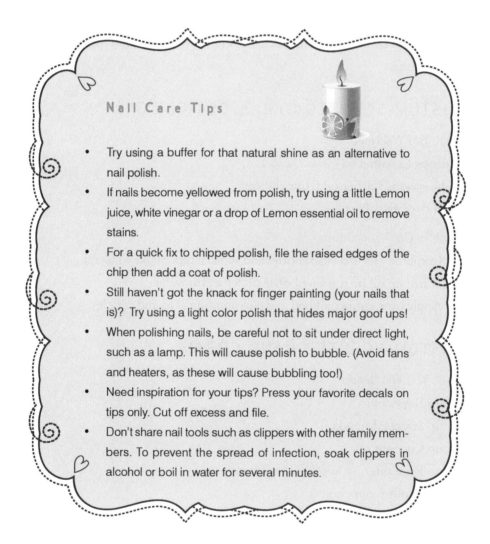

Nail Care Tips

- Try using a buffer for that natural shine as an alternative to nail polish.
- If nails become yellowed from polish, try using a little Lemon juice, white vinegar or a drop of Lemon essential oil to remove stains.
- For a quick fix to chipped polish, file the raised edges of the chip then add a coat of polish.
- Still haven't got the knack for finger painting (your nails that is)? Try using a light color polish that hides major goof ups!
- When polishing nails, be careful not to sit under direct light, such as a lamp. This will cause polish to bubble. (Avoid fans and heaters, as these will cause bubbling too!)
- Need inspiration for your tips? Press your favorite decals on tips only. Cut off excess and file.
- Don't share nail tools such as clippers with other family members. To prevent the spread of infection, soak clippers in alcohol or boil in water for several minutes.

Essential Oils for Hands and Feet

CUTICLE OILS Add up to 30 drops of essential oil per 2 ounces carrier oil. Be sure to check the potency of the essential oils before adding. With stronger essential oils your blend will require considerably less. Always use more carrier oil than essential oils. The general rule of thumb for blending cuticle oils is 3%-10% essential oil and 90%-97% carrier oil.

NAIL CUTICLE SOAKS For single use, add 1 cup of water, 1 tablespoon carrier oil, and up to 15 drops of essential oils to a small bowl.

FOOT SOAKS In a foot bath or tub, add up to 30 drops of essential oils.

BOOST NAIL GROWTH Essential oils that help boost nail growth includes: Evening Primrose, Lavender, Lemon, Tea Tree, Patchouli,

Sandalwood, and Equisetum arvense (Horsetail).

NAIL FUNGUS Essential oils for treating nail fungus includes: Tea Tree, Oregano, Thyme, Clove, Ravensara, Lemongrass, Frankincense, Myrrh, Lavender, and Flu Buster blend.

WEAK NAILS Essential oils good for weak nails includes: Frankincense, Myrrh, and Lemon.

SOFTEN CUTICLES Essential oils that help soften cuticles includes: Eucalyptus and Peppermint.

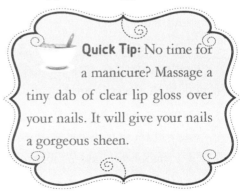

Quick Tip: No time for a manicure? Massage a tiny dab of clear lip gloss over your nails. It will give your nails a gorgeous sheen.

HOME SALON MANICURE

You don't have to go to a sophisticated salon for that polished look. You can do-it-yourself as your own home manicurist. Here's how!

What You Will Need:

Hand Towel

Warm Water

Small Bowl

Nail Clippers

Nail Brush

Nail Polish

Nail Polish Remover

Cotton Pads (or balls)

Orange Stick (or a popsicle stick)

Emery Board

Cuticle Cream or oil

Mild Facial Cleanser (or moisturizing soap)

Moisturizing Hand Lotion

2 tablespoons Olive oil

What To Do:

1. Remove old nail polish by wetting a cotton pad with nail polish remover and holding on nails for a few seconds, allowing nail polish to dissolve. Then, wipe away in sweeping motion outward to keep cuticles and skin clean.

2. Wash your hands with moisturizing soap and warm water. Pat hands dry with a hand towel.

3. Clip nails to a length slightly longer than what you want (mid to short length is ideal).

4. File with emery board to get nails to desired length. File from the outer corners toward the tip. Do not use a "sawing" motion (back and forth); this will cause nails to become jagged.

5. In a small bowl, add 2 tablespoons of olive oil to warm water and soak hands for 5-10 minutes.

6. Clean nails with a nail brush, then apply cuticle cream to the cuticles. Massage hands with moisturizing hand lotion, using your thumb in a circular motion.

7. Using your orange stick, gently push back cuticles. Then, wipe hands again using your hand towel to remove excess lotion.

8. Take your nail polish and apply at the center of the nail with one stroke. Then, apply two more strokes on either side to cover nail. Be careful to only have enough polish on the brush for one stroke at a time. Allow 1-2 minutes to dry before applying second coat.

9. Allow nails to dry completely. To speed up drying time, dip fingers into a bowl of icy water for a couple of minutes after your final coat. Air dry.

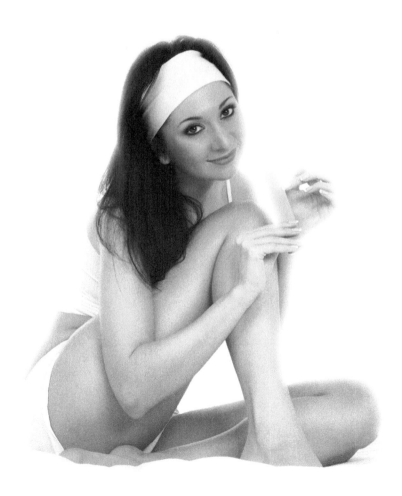

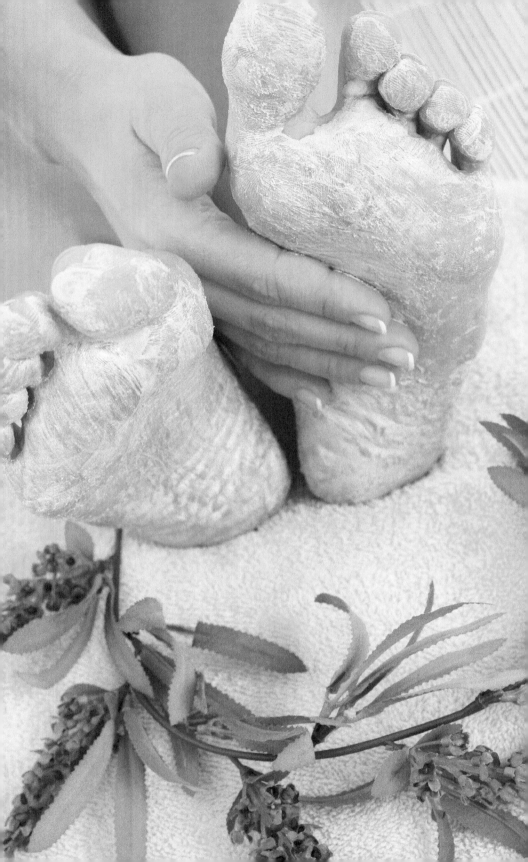

Essential Care for the Feet

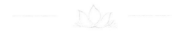

No matter if you're barefoot and pregnant or stepping out on the town in platform heels, we all rely on our feet to carry us everywhere and even dance the night away! You probably don't give them much thought until a problem develops like a bunion, callus, or corn.

Now you can give your achy feet a break and rejuvenate them with essential oils. The natural effects of the oils can help treat your feet when they are tired, sore, cracked or just simply worn out. In this chapter, you will find all the treats your feet deserve: foot scrubs, foot baths, foot lotions, foot powders and more.

It's time now to get those toes ready for flip flops. Jump in and get your feet wet with some of these recipes!

BEACH SAND FOOT SCRUB

What You Will Need:

2 tablespoons Canola oil

2 tablespoons Beach Sand

3-5 drops Rosemary essential oil

What To Do:

1. Combine all of the ingredients and mix into a paste.
2. Massage scrub onto feet, concentrating especially on problem areas. Rinse off with warm water and pat feet dry.

ALOE-OATMEAL FOOT SCRUB

What You Will Need:

¼ cup Unscented Organic Lotion

¼ cup Oatmeal, finely grounded

¼ cup Cornmeal

¼ cup Sea Salt

2 tablespoons Aloe Vera gel

What To Do:

1. In a bowl, mix all of the ingredients together to form a paste.
2. To use, massage into the feet then rinse well.

BROWN SUGAR EXFOLIATING FOOT SCRUB

What You Will Need:

2 tablespoons Brown Sugar

1 tablespoon Lemon juice

1 tablespoon Honey

1 teaspoon Olive oil

2 tablespoons Oatmeal, finely grounded

Essential oils

Jar

What To Do:

1. In a bowl, add all of the ingredients and stir.
2. Add 10-20 drops of your favorite essential oils and blend well.
3. Pour the mixture into a small wide-mouth glass jar or a 4-ounce plastic salve container.
4. To use the scrub, place a small amount in the palm and scrub over moist-ened skin and rough patches. Rinse off in a shower or tub.

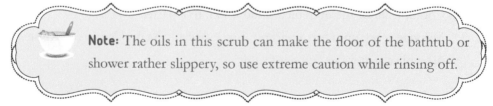

Note: The oils in this scrub can make the floor of the bathtub or shower rather slippery, so use extreme caution while rinsing off.

SEA SALT FOOT SCRUB

What You Will Need:

1 cup Sea Salt

¼ cup Cornmeal

¼ cup Sweet Almond oil

10 drops Spearmint essential oil

What To Do:

1. In a bowl, combine all of the ingredients.
2. To use, rub over heels and rough patches. Rinse with water.

SOOTHING CRACKED FEET MASK

What You Will Need:

1 cup Rolled Oats

½ cup Flour

¼ cup Honey

¼ cup Olive oil

10 drops Lavender essential oil

5 drops Tea Tree essential oil

Baking Soda

What You Will Need:

1. In a bowl, mix all of the ingredients and stir well. It will have a sticky consistency. If too dry, add a little more oil.
2. Soak feet in a foot tub of warm water and baking soda for 10 minutes before using foot mask.
3. Apply foot mask to feet and leave on for 20-30 minutes. Rinse off and dry feet. Apply moisturizer if desired.

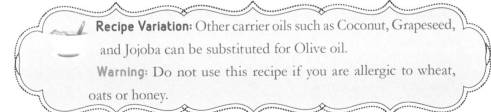

Recipe Variation: Other carrier oils such as Coconut, Grapeseed, and Jojoba can be substituted for Olive oil.

Warning: Do not use this recipe if you are allergic to wheat, oats or honey.

CITRUS FOOT MASSAGE BAR

Give your favorite person a foot massage with this bar or give yourself one!

What You Will Need:

4 tablespoons Solid Vegetable Shortening

3 tablespoons Solid Cocoa butter

2 tablespoons Solid Coconut oil

1 tablespoon Beeswax

1 tablespoon Soy Wax

10 drops Orange essential oil (or whatever you like)

1-3 drops Natural Orange Food Coloring

Mold

Cooking spray

What To Do:

1. Spray mold with cooking spray to prevent sticking.

2. Add all of the ingredients except the essential oil and natural food coloring in a microwave safe dish and heat for 3 minutes (or use a double boiler on the stovetop). Stir until liquefied.

3. Add the natural food coloring. Beat for several minutes until emulsified and slightly thick. If it isn't thickening, place your bowl in ice water as you beat it with an electric mixer.

4. Add essential oil. Pour into molds. Refrigerate until set.

5. Wrap in plastic and store in a cool place. To use, simply hand warm your molded oil before use.

ENERGIZING FOOT LOTION

This lotion is good for when you have been on your feet all day and want something soothing.

What You Will Need:

1 tablespoon Sweet Almond oil

1 tablespoon Olive oil

1 teaspoon Wheat Germ oil

12 drops Eucalyptus essential oil

What To Do:

1. Combine all of the ingredients in a bottle and shake to blend well.

2. To use, rub into the feet and heels. Store in a cool, dry place.

BANANA FOOT CREAM

Dry feet will become smooth overnight when you use this cream.

What You Will Need:

½ Banana

1 tablespoon Honey

3 drops Lemon essential oil

1 tablespoon Sweet Almond oil

What To Do:

1. Mix all of the ingredients together.

2. Smear on feet and wear thick socks to bed. Wash off in the morning.

STRAWBERRY-ALMOND FOOT CREAM

Smooth rough edges with this foot cream!

What You Will Need:

8 Strawberries

2 tablespoons Olive oil

1 teaspoon Sea Salt

1 teaspoon Finely Chopped Almonds

2 drops Vanilla essential oil

What To Do:

1. Mix all of the ingredients thoroughly.

2. Massage over the feet and then rinse off with warm water. Dry feet.

COOL GINGER FOOT POWDER

This light, fragrant powder absorbs moisture and fights bacteria to eradicate perspiration and body odor. It also helps relieve Athlete's foot. Both Tea Tree and Ginger have antiseptic and antifungal properties.

What You Will Need:

½ cup Arrowroot, powdered

½ cup White Clay

2 tablespoons Ginger, powdered

20 drops Tea Tree essential oil

What To Do:

1. In a large jar, combine the arrowroot, cosmetic clay and Ginger. Cover and shake to mix.
2. Add Tea Tree essential oil and shake again.
3. Sift the powder through a fine mesh strainer to break up any drops of oil.
4. Store in a covered, dark glass jar. Apply as needed to feet or body. The powder will keep indefinitely.

HAPPY FEET POWDER

Keep feet happy and dry by using this powder on your feet and inside shoes.

What You Will Need:

2 tablespoons Corn Flour

15 drops Lavender essential oil

5 drops Tea Tree essential oil

Small plastic bag

What To Do:

1. Add corn flour into a small plastic bag.
2. Add the essential oils to the mixture.
3. Close bag and allow it to sit for 24 hours. Shake well before using.

PEPPERMINT FOOT MASSAGE OIL

Your toes will love the minty, refreshing feeling!

What You Will Need:

10 teaspoons Grapeseed oil

3 drops Eucalyptus essential oil

4 drops Rosemary essential oil

2 drops Peppermint essential oil

Small dark glass bottle

What To Do:

1. Combine oils in a small bottle.
2. Warm up oil before doing any foot massage by running under warm water.

KILLER ANTI-FUNGAL OIL

Oregano essential oil works well as a powerful antiseptic and fungicide. This one will save you a trip to the doctor with this effective at-home treatment for conditions such as nail fungus and Athlete's foot.

What You Will Need:

2 drops Oregano essential oil

1 teaspoon Olive oil

Small dark glass bottle

What To Do:

1. Add Olive oil and Oregano essential oil to a small bottle. Shake well to mix.
2. Rub on afflicted area every day for a maximum of 3 weeks.

SAGE DEODORIZING FOOT POWDER

What You Will Need:

1 tablespoon Baking Powder

2 drops Sage essential oil

Plastic Bag

What To Do:

1. Mix baking powder and oil in a plastic bag and shake well.
2. Allow to dry. Break up any clumps that may have formed.
3. Dust feet regularly with the powder and add a teaspoon in the shoes overnight.

LEMON FOOT SOAK

Great for dry, rough feet!

What You Will Need:

1 bowl Warm Water

1 Lemon juice

4 drops Lemon essential oil

What To Do:

1. In a bowl, add Lemon juice and Lemon essential oil to warm water.
2. Soak feet for 15-20 minutes.

MUSTARD FOOT BATH

What You Will Need:

½ cup Baking Soda

2 tablespoons Mustard Powder

2 drops Rosemary essential oil

2 drops Tea Tree essential oil

Jar or container with lid

What To Do:

1. In a bowl or basin, combine all of the ingredients.
2. Add two tablespoons of mixture to hot water and soak feet for 15 minutes.
3. Store in a jar or container until ready to use.

SAGE FOOT BATH

What You Will Need:

Warm Water

2 drops Sage essential oil

What To Do:

1. Add 2 drops of Sage essential oil to a foot tub or basin of warm water.
2. Soak your feet in a bowl with this mixture every day for a week.

TEA TREE & LAVENDER FOOT FUNGUS SOAK

Try nature's holistic approach to healing before running out to the drug store
to purchase over-the-counter medicines for nail fungus.

What You Will Need:

1 cup Apple Cider vinegar, warmed

6 drops Tea Tree essential oil

6 drops Lavender essential oil

1 cup Warm Water

Bowl or foot basin

What To Do:

1. Blend ingredients into a large bowl.
2. Soak for 10-20 minutes several times a week to kill fungus.

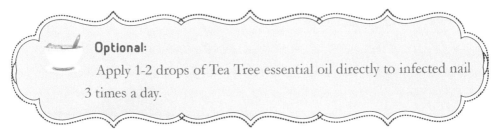

Optional:
Apply 1-2 drops of Tea Tree essential oil directly to infected nail
3 times a day.

CUSTOM-SCENTED FOOT POWDER

What You Will Need:

1 tablespoon Baking Powder

2 drops Essential oil (your choice)

Plastic Bag

What To Do:

1. Mix baking powder and oil in a plastic bag and shake well.
2. Allow to dry. Break up any clumps that may have formed.
3. Dust feet regularly with the powder and add a teaspoon in the shoes overnight.

CUSTOM-SCENTED FOOT SCRUB

What You Will Need:

¼ cup Sea Salt or Sugar

¼ cup Carrier oil (Coconut, Jojoba, Sweet Almond, or Olive)

10-12 drops Essential oil (your choice)

Wide-mouth Jar

What To Do:

1. In a bowl or wide-mouth jar, add the sea salt or sugar. Pour in the carrier oil of your choice. Stir to mix.
2. Add your favorite essential oil into the wet mixture and stir to blend well.
3. To use, place a small amount of the scrub in the palm of your hand and rub over moistened feet while showering or taking a bath. Rinse off.

Recipe Variation:

Add a couple of Vitamin E capsules for added health benefits.

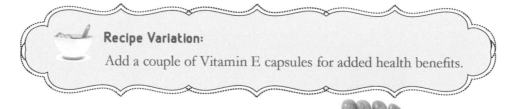

Feet Care Tips

- Use a Loofah sponge to exfoliate the top, sides and bottoms of your feet. After drying your feet, apply a creamy moisturizer and wear thick soft socks to bed.

- Be careful to not slip or fall when using your foot scrub in the shower or tub, as it can make the floor slippery. Be sure to rinse excess oils off well.

- Wash your feet on a regular basis to prevent fungal infection between your toes. Not only does this cause bad foot odor, it itches and causes dry, flaky skin.

- Always wear clean socks. When feet get wet from perspiration, change socks and/or remove shoes to let feet breathe.

- Use leftover foot scrub on other rough skin areas, such as the knees or elbows.

- Store unused foot scrubs in the refrigerator and use within 3 weeks.

- Blisters are caused by skin friction. Don't pop them. Keep your feet dry—wear socks as a cushion between your feet and shoes. If a blister breaks, wash the area, apply an antiseptic essential oil such as Tea Tree or Lavender and cover with a sterile bandage.

- Prevent ingrown nails by trimming toenails straight across and slightly longer than the end of the toe with toenail clippers. Always wear shoes that fit properly and won't cause pressure on the corners of nails digging painfully into the skin. Use your emery board to smooth rough edges.

- Don't ignore foot pain—it's not normal. If the pain persists, see a podiatric physician.

- Soak your feet in lukewarm water with essential oil regularly to ease tiredness and get rid of your body's toxins.

- Before stepping out in the sun, make sure you have applied a generous amount of sunscreen on your feet as well.

- Foot powders are the best way to soak up excessive moisture during the hot months. This will help you stay refreshed the entire day and ease you from the trouble of smelly feet.

Feet Care Tips (continues)

- Remove calluses or tough worn patches of skin by using a pumice stone. To prevent getting calluses on the feet, wear cotton socks.

- For warmer weather when toes are exposed, you will want to give yourself a weekly pedicure. Follow the same directions as for the *Home Salon Manicure.*

- Feet and legs have little or no oil glands so you will need to moisturize twice as often as you do for your hands. The best time to do this is after a bath for faster absorption.

- Popular essential oils to use on the feet include: Peppermint for its anti-inflammatory properties, Lavender for its soothing and relaxing effects, Rosemary's stimulating properties for aches and pains, and Lemon and Eucalyptus for their antiviral and antiseptic properties.

- Before doing a pedicure, start with an aromatherapy foot bath to soften calluses and make toenails pliable. Foot baths are also great for relieving aches, pains, tiredness and burning feet.

- If you suffer from athlete's foot or another fungal infection, try using these essential oils: Peppermint, Geranium, Sage, Tea Tree, Thyme, Myrrh, Clove, and Lemon.

- To administer a foot massage, use circular motions focusing on the ball of the foot to relieve stress and induce relaxation.

Index

Y

Photo Credits

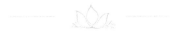

Aromatherapy.Spa Collection ©iStockphoto.com/VikZa

Soaps Stacked Isolated ©iStockphoto.com/Mishooo

Relaxation Spa Concept ©iStockphoto.com/NightandDayImages

Foot Skincare, Skin Scrubbing ©iStockphoto.com/Beemore

Shea butter and nuts in bowl ©iStockphoto.com/Elenathewise

Cute woman doing manicure on the white bed ©iStockphoto.com/Osuleo

Bottles of Spa Oil and Salt ©iStockphoto.com/Tpopova

Natural homemade organic facial masks of honey ©iStockphoto.com/Targovcom

Natural Homemade Facial Masks ©iStockphoto.com/Targovcom

Girl Getting a Shampoo ©iStockphoto.com/Stockphoto4u

Foot-Care ©iStockphoto.com/ Matka_Wariatka

Spa Icons ©iStockphoto.com/LumpyNoodles

Spa Isolated ©iStockphoto.com/Bluehill75

Toilet Soap ©Popova Olga – Fotolia.com

Milk Powder with water ©Grasko – Fotolia.com

Fresh Honeycombs ©Sergejs Rahunoks – Fotolia.com

Woman's Foot into Foam Bath with Painted Fingernails © saap585 – Fotolia.com

Woman Removing Makeup © studiovespa - Fotolia.com

Beauty-spa Applying Mud Mask © volff - Fotolia.com

Massage Oils and Lotus Flower © MAXFX - Fotolia.com

Happy Woman Taking Milk Bath © Dmytro Konstantynov - Fotolia.com

Bomb © mrs. Blondy - Fotolia.com

Set of Retro Vignettes © MariykaA - Fotolia.com

Other Books by
Rebecca Park Totilo

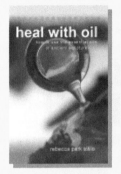

HEAL WITH OIL: HOW TO USE THE ESSENTIAL OILS OF ANCIENT SCRIPTURE

God has provided a natural remedy to our Healthcare crisis - essential oils extracted from plants and trees. In this practical guide, Rebecca instructs believers on how to use the twelve healing oils mentioned in Holy Scriptures for healing and restoration of the body. Learn about the hidden treasures of the Levitical Priests and what the pharmaceutical companies don't want you to know. Book includes practical advice on blending oils and safety, a directory of properties for twelve oils from the Bible and special blends for the bath and personal care. Tons of recipes for beauty, health and emotional well-being.

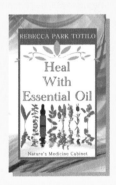

HEAL WITH ESSENTIAL OIL: NATURE'S MEDICINE CABINET

Using essential oils drawn from nature's own medicine cabinet of flowers, trees, seeds and roots, man can tap into God's healing power to heal oneself from almost any pain. Find relief from many conditions and rejuvenate the body. With over 125 recipes, this practical guide will walk you through in the most easy-to-understand form how to treat common ailments with your essential oils for everyday living. Filled with practical advice on therapeutic blending of oils and safety, a directory of the most effective oils for common ailments and easy to follow remedies chart and prescriptive blends for aches, pains and sicknesses.

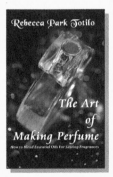

THE ART OF MAKING PERFUME

With a ton of recipes and helpful hints on perfume making, you'll discover how to make homemade perfumes, body sprays, aftershave colognes, floral waters and much more using pure essential oils. Rebecca shares insider secrets from the beauty industry how to develop your very own signature fragrance. Topics include: History of Perfumery, The Ancient Art of Extracting Oils & Making Perfumes, Easy-to-Follow Steps on Perfume Making, Perfumes for Holistic Healing & Well-Being, Perfumes Kids Can Make, Perfume For Your Dog, & How to Start Your Own Perfume Business.

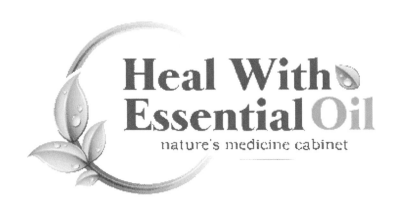

For other books, DVDs, and essential oils products,
please visit our website:
http://HealWithEssentialOil.com

For e-mail correspondence, please write:
info@healwithessentialoil.com

For snail mail correspondence:
Heal With Essential Oil
P.O. Box 60044
St. Petersburg, FL 33784

CPSIA information can be obtained at www.ICGtesting.com
Printed in the USA
LVOW010713240413

330676LV00014B/51/P